HEALING MUDRAS
FOR YOUR SOUL

VOLUME III.

NEW REVISED
FULL COLOR EDITION

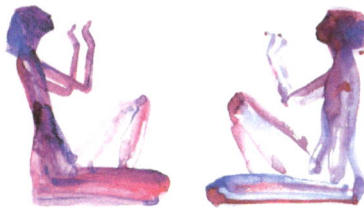

SABRINA MESKO PH.D.H.

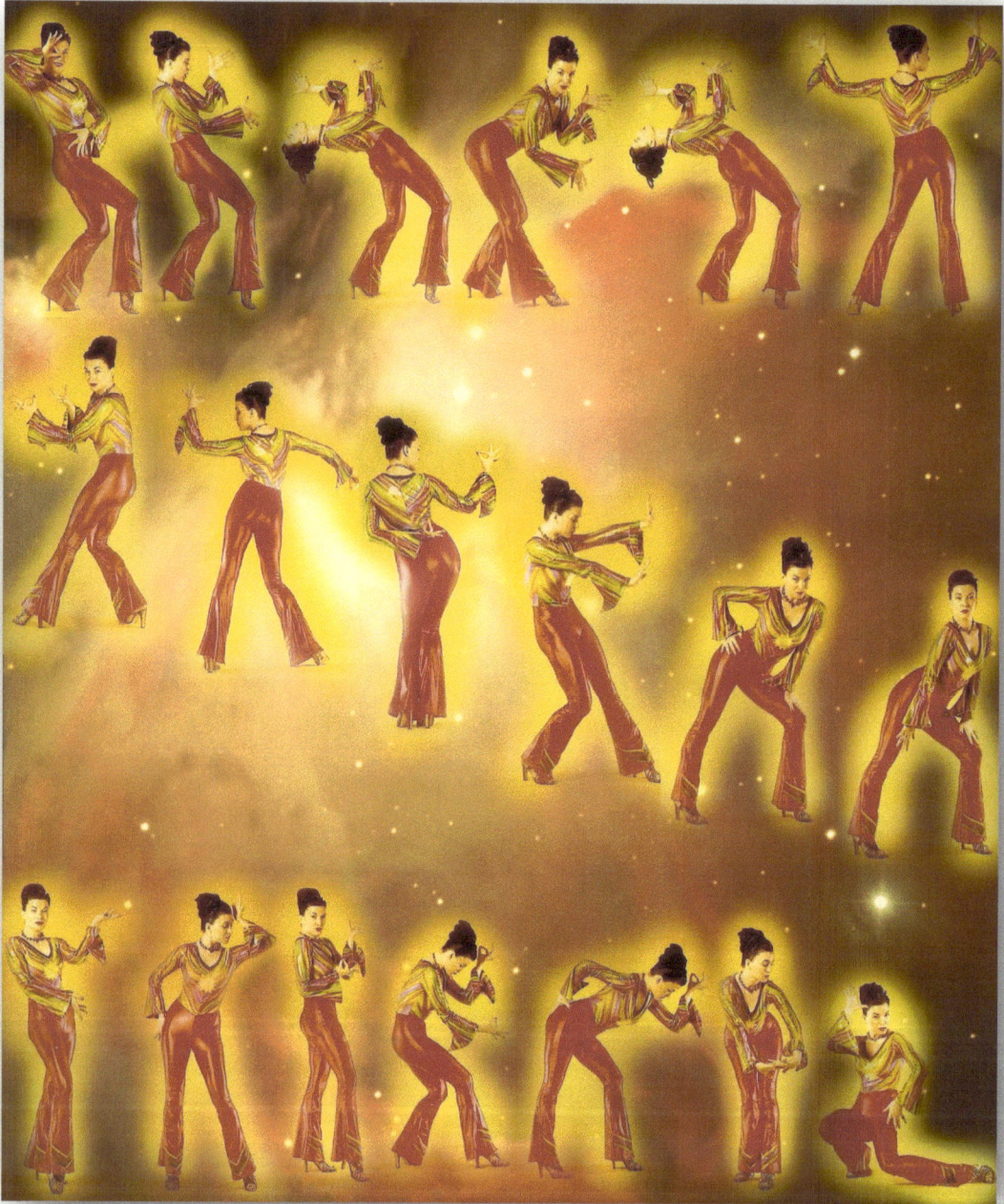

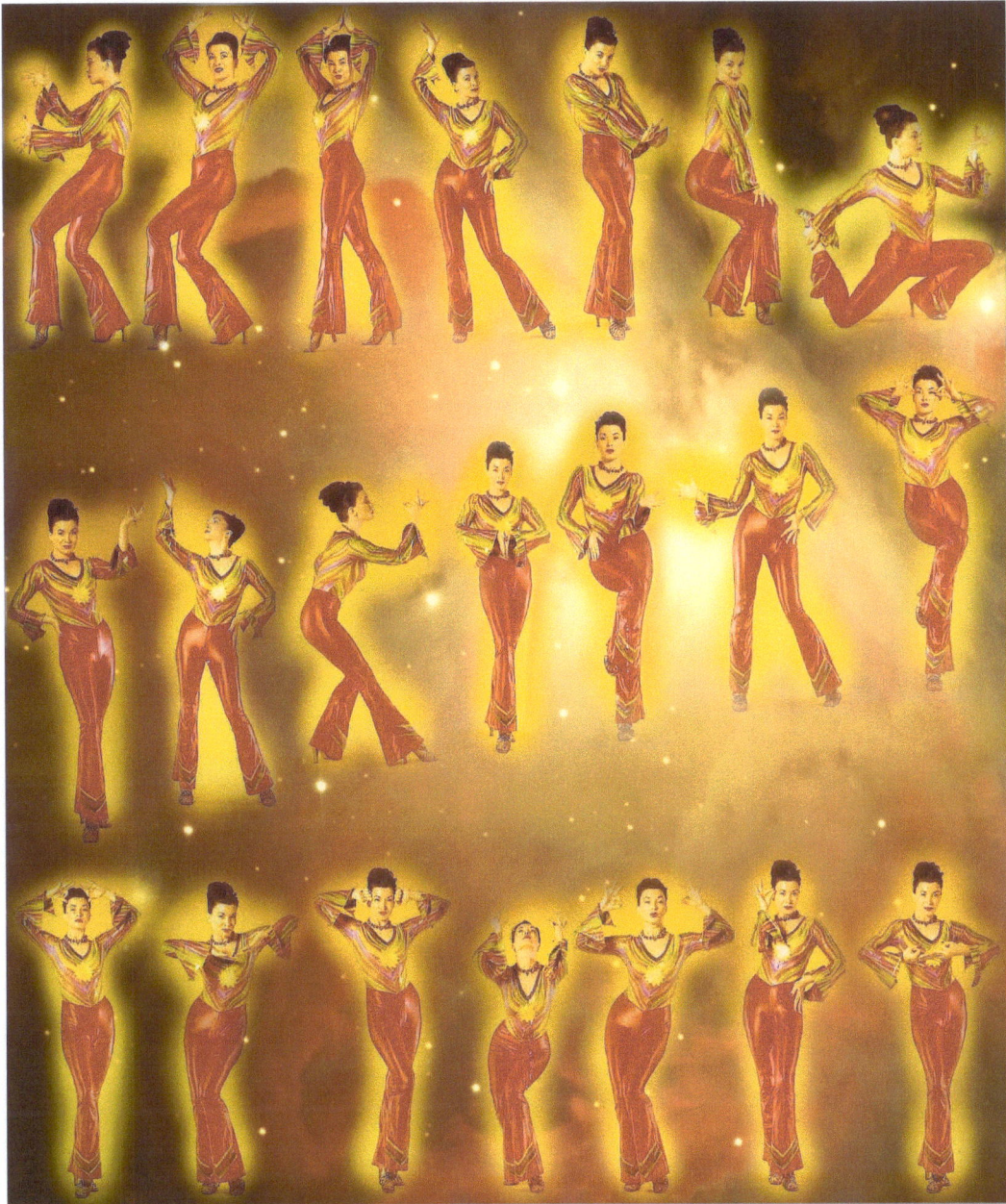

The material contained in this book is not intended as medical advice.
If you have a medical issue or illness, consult a qualified physician.

A Mudra Hands™ Book
Published by Mudra Hands Publishing

Photography by Dorothy Low
Illustrations by Kiar Mesko
Costume design, photo design, and styling by Sabrina Mesko
Cover photo by Dorothy Low
On The Cover ~ MUDRA for Contentment

Printed in the United States of America

ISBN-13: 978-0615810881
ISBN-10: 0615810888

Originally published by Random House in 2000
Under the title *Healing Mudras -Yoga for Your Hands*
New, revised, updated and expanded

To the greatest parents in the world,
Bibi and Kiar

BY SABRINA MESKO

HEALING MUDRAS
Yoga for Your Hands
Random House - Original edition

POWER MUDRAS
Yoga Hand Postures for Women
Random House - Original edition

MUDRA - GESTURES OF POWER
DVD - Sounds True

CHAKRA MUDRAS DVD set
HAND YOGA for Vitality, Creativity and Success
HAND YOGA for Concentration, Love and Longevity

HEALING MUDRAS
Yoga for Your Hands - New Edition

HEALING MUDRAS - New Edition in full color:
Healing Mudras I. ~ For Your Body
Healing Mudras II. ~ For Your Mind
Healing Mudras III. ~ For Your Soul

POWER MUDRAS
Yoga Hand Postures for Women - New Edition

MUDRA THERAPY
Hand Yoga for Pain Management and Conquering Illness

YOGA MIND
45 Meditations for Inner Peace, Prosperity and Protection

MUDRAS FOR ASTROLOGICAL SIGNS
Volumes I. ~ XII.

MUDRAS FOR ARIES, TAURUS, GEMINI, CANCER, LEO, VIRGO, LIBRA, SCORPIO, SAGITTARIUS, CAPRICORN, AQUARIUS, PISCES
12 Book Series

LOVE MUDRAS
Hand Yoga for Two

MUDRAS AND CRYSTALS
The Alchemy of Energy Protection

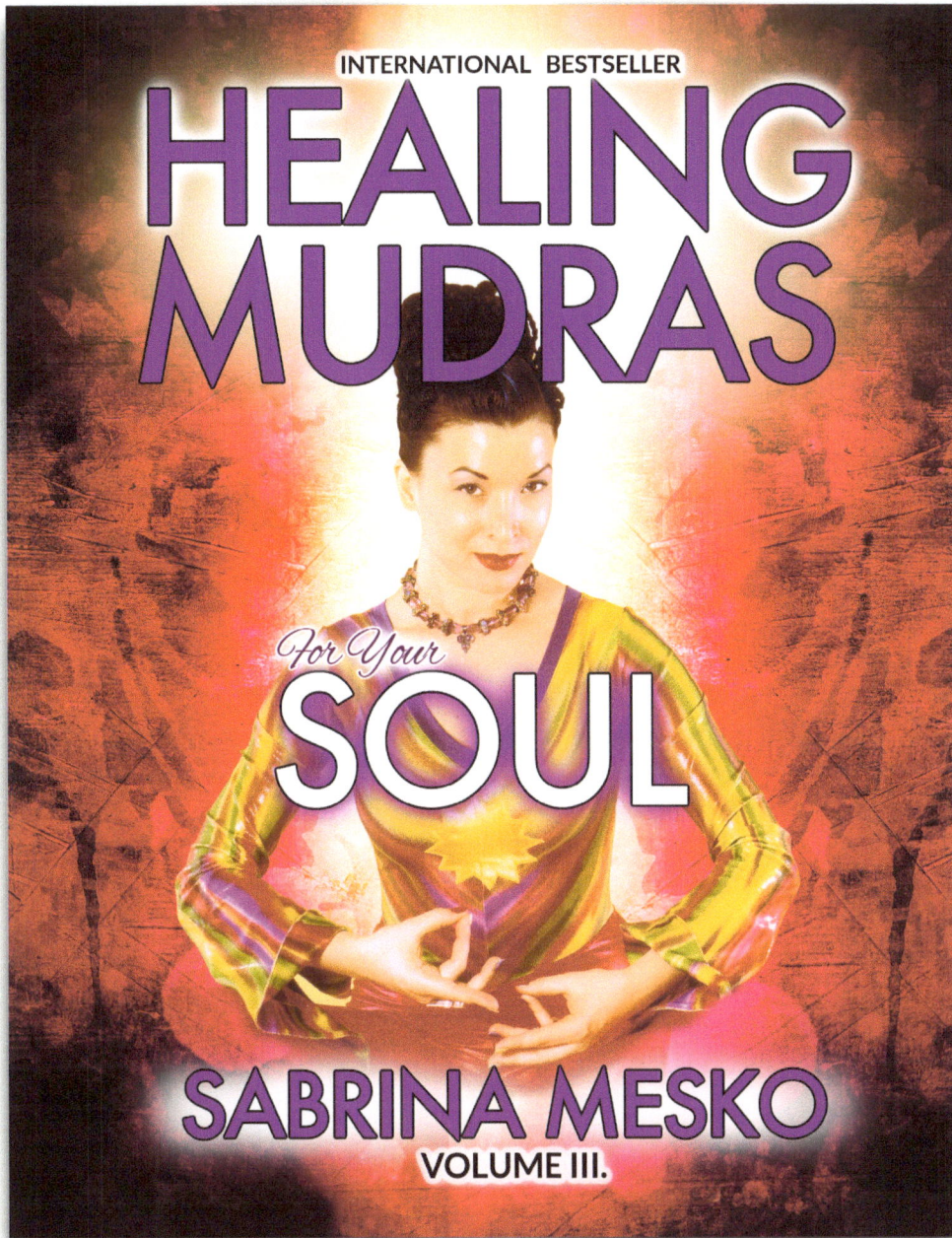

INTERNATIONAL BESTSELLER

HEALING MUDRAS

For Your

SOUL

SABRINA MESKO
VOLUME III.

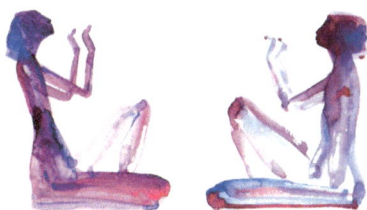

CONTENTS

MUDRAS FOR YOUR SOUL

HEALING MUDRAS
FOR
YOUR SOUL

YOGA FOR YOUR HANDS

INTRODUCTION

Mudras are the ancient sacred codes to your body, mind and spirit. They are a part of your everyday lives, intuitively used and intricately affecting your energy level, self-healing capacity and energy reception and output. The healing powers of Mudras are undeniable and needed now more than ever.

Thirteen years have passed since the original HEALING MUDRAS was published. As every author will tell you, the moment you let the book out of your hands, it begins a life of its own. Whether it is a long life or a short one, it depends on so many factors. HEALING MUDRAS is long-lived, for it has been translated into over 14 languages and has positively affected thousands of Mudra practitioners around the world. Since the first publication, I have traveled the globe, taught people these powerful ancient techniques in different languages, and received countless letters of gratitude for bringing Mudras into today's spotlight. Every time I receive a reader's letter, I am deeply joyful that another person has benefited from these techniques, and humbled for the opportunity of being a part of that process. I am only the messenger and instrument to convey these ancient sacred Mudras. It is truly a part of my life's mission and an honor to have had the pleasure of teaching Mudras to all kinds of audiences, all ages, all cultures, religions and spiritual convictions, or openness to healing aspects of such practices. I can honestly say that each and every person who practiced Mudras, has experienced the power magnitude of positive effects. It has been an amazing journey that continues to this day.

Mudras will always be a profound part of my life, and since the readers have asked me numerous times when my next project will be released, I have created a double DVD series titled Chakra Mudras to help expand available practice materials. And now the time has come for an updated NEW edition HEALING MUDRAS - a new revised version of the first book with the additional chapter. I have decided to offer the reader two choices; a complete book with black and white photographs, and a color version of the book in three separate volumes, for Body, Mind and Soul. The color edition was my original wish for the look and feel of the book and is now realized. What you hold in your hands is the Volume III. with full color photographs, nevertheless you, my dear reader, have the choice.

My early years as a professional ballerina left within me a permanent imprint of discipline and persistence and I apply that to every aspect of my work with Mudras. They are such precise and intricate hand positions that need to be practiced with accuracy and focus to produce optimal results.

You have to be present, truly immerse yourself into the Mudra practice and then....most wondrous things happen. Mudras take charge and you can follow your hands and experience the true depth of these ancient codes. Suddenly your soul power unlocks and is set free, your life perspective changes and you understand and perceive this earthly experience in a deeper, more profound way, all the while with a healthy distance from challenging times and expanded understanding of fortunate ones.

Each lifetime seems to have a hidden pendulum that swings back and forth, it seems there is an invisible balance that remains, no matter how it all appears to others from the outside. There is an order, there is a purpose and there is a designated path that each one of us is on, but all of our life's mysteries cannot be revealed at once. We must remain attentive in the present, the now, to truly experience every nuance that this earthly incarnation offers to teach us. If we understand and respect the pendulum, the balance will remain intact. If we fight it, it will be thrown off.

The inner balance is the true key to be able to journey thru life with enduring vigor and loving generosity while surrendering the final outcome to the invisible universal power that resides in us all. We must trust this universal navigation, for it knows us better than we ever will. It loves us more than we ever will. And it has a better plan for us than we could ever imagine. Mudras are one of these sacred keys, for they are connected to your every move and every breath. Understand them, use them, and let them serve you on your way to enlightenment, self-realization, healing, and the absolute fulfillment of your optimal potential.

As always, I remain eternally grateful for being given the opportunity to be the instrument for the transmission of these sacred teachings to you.

One in Spirit, love, and Peace. Blessings to all,

Sabrina

THE HISTORY AND ART OF MUDRA

Hand gestures have been native to every culture on earth and can be seen as intrinsic to civilization: Ancient Egyptians, Romans, Greeks, Persians, Aborigines in Australia, ancient Indians and Chinese, Africans, Turks, Fijians, Mayan cultures, Inuit, and the Native American nations all used hand gestures.

Today, we still use hand language. Think about the universal handshake — a sign of friendship and peace. Applause is the language for approval and enthusiasm; the pointed index finger is used to scold; an upraised hand with the palm -out signals us to stop.

There are many points of view regarding the development of hand gestures. Scientists have proved that even apes communicate with their hands and firmly believe that hand gestures were basis for speech. A blind child who has never been able to see will still clap his hands to express excitement and happiness. Many hand gestures are universal, dating back thousands of years. In Egypt almost five thousand years ago, hand gestures were performed in prayer rituals by high priests and priestesses. Sacred hand gestures were key to communicating with the gods, manifesting miracles, and connecting with the afterlife. Egyptians carved these sacred gestures in bas-reliefs on the walls of and inside the pyramids, and they became the basis for their hieroglyphs. From Egypt these movements and knowledge of their spiritual power and usage traveled to India and Greece.

In India, these gestures were named "mudras," a Sanskrit word, and they became an irreplaceable part of yoga, which aimed to connect the practitioner to divine and cosmic energy. Mudras became the essence of this divine communication in Buddhism and Hinduism. Buddhist priests developed the understanding of mudras still further and used them to close prayer rituals, a practice that has remained alive to this day.

Plato placed hand gestures among the civil virtues in ancient Greece, where there was a distinct classification of hand gestures into comic, tragic, and satiric. From Egypt and Greece, these hand gestures were brought to Rome, where they became intrinsic to popular discourse and culture.

In the reign of Emperor Augustus in Rome, performances of hand gestures in pantomimic dances were a great personal delight of the emperor. Competitions were held between the best hand – gesture dancers, and all Rome was split into factions about their favorites. The most distinguished performer was often called the Dancing Philosopher.

In the year 190, there were six thousand performers in Rome devoted to the art of hand gesture. Their popularity continued until the sixth century A.D. Sacred hand gestures were also used in religious practice among Jews. In various portrayals of Moses we can observe him using mudras with gestures of blessing, divine protection, knowledge, and receiving guidance from the divine.

In Christianity, mudras took on a less noticeable form. Stylized hand poses are almost always present in portrayals of Jesus, but most people were not taught the significance of these poses. So the people in Western cultures lost the awareness of the healing and sacred power of the mudras and used them more as expressive communication gestures.

In Italian paintings before and during the renaissance, one of the most common hand poses is that of the connected thumb and index finger. Its meaning is that the ego – the index finger – is bowing to God – the thumb – in love and unity. In popular Neapolitan use, that gesture is called the kissing of the thumb and finger – the sign of love. In secular portraits, that gesture translates into approval of love and marriage. Some Native Americans also used that hand gesture when indicating that they thought something was good and approved of it.

Another common gesture in religious paintings is that of the palm turned upward. This pose dates back centuries and signifies openness and inquiry. In this book, it is part of the mudra of asking for guidance, and it has a part in mudra for facing fear. When you ask the Universe to protect and guide you, the palm is held so that something can be placed in your hand – something can come to you. American Indians translated this gesture into: Give me!

A gesture in which the pointed index finger moves in a circle has a universal connection – specifically, "no" – rejection in Italian, native American, and Japanese cultures, among others. When the index finger is pointed but motionless in popular usage and in high Italian art, it means indication, justice, pointing something out (which has led to the actual name of index for the forefinger). It can also mean silence, attention, number, mediation, and demonstration. Native Americans were among the most famed hand – sign communicators, usually signing in front of strangers. Early white settles actually believed that the American Indians rarely used spoken language, since the settlers most often saw them using hand gestures that Europeans didn't understand. Later on, Native Americans would play a key role in communicating with hearing – impaired children.

In Mexico, hand signs are found in elaborate ancient carvings, and they are also painted on ancient Greek and Homeric vases and pottery writings. The Chinese alphabet actually originated as the depiction of hand gestures. There are many commonalities among the hand gestures of Native American, Chinese, Egyptian, and African cultures. I hope that archeologists, anthropologists, and linguists can eventually piece together how these universal gestures come to be used in such different parts of the world. Hand gestures are the mother of all communication and are supremely powerful. The art of mudra is divinely inspired: It enables us to communicate with the divine, develop and aspire to higher qualities, and keep a universally popular language. Mudra is our connection to the divine play of the cosmos.

The time has come to revive and appreciate the gift of mudras practice to utilize these efficient, powerful ancient techniques in your everyday life. Mudra can help you follow your dreams: Your life is in your hands. There are no limitations.

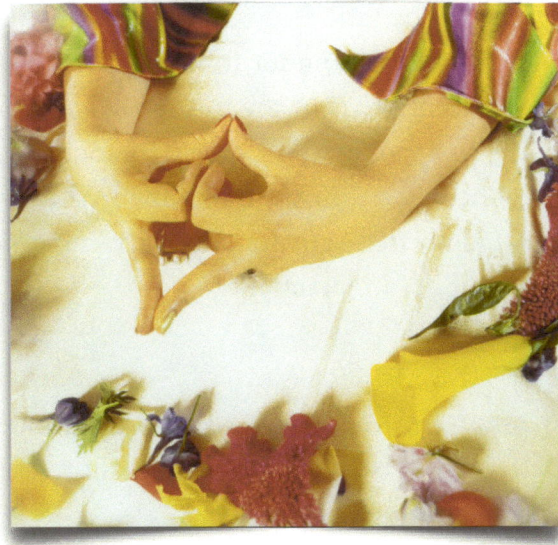

MUDRA FOR TRANQUILIZING YOUR MIND

THE PRACTICE OF MUDRA

INSTRUCTIONS FOR PRACTICE

WHERE DO I PRACTICE MUDRA?

To practice mudra, find a quiet, peaceful, and private place where no one can disturb you. If that is not always possible, you can usually practice most of the mudras that are unobtrusive just about anywhere.

HOW DO I PRACTICE MUDRA?

During the practice, it is best to sit in a comfortable position. You can sit on a pillow or blanket in a cross-legged position, or in a chair, but make sure your weight on both feet is equal. It is most important that you keep your back straight. Maintain a comfortable sitting posture that does *not* give you pain.

WHEN SHOULD I PRACTICE MUDRA?

You can practice a mudra virtually any time that you feel the need to connect with the energy that it gives you. If you are practicing a mudra for insight or to enhance your meditation, however, the easiest time to concentrate is in the morning right after you wake up or in the evening before going to sleep. You should never practice a mudra on a full stomach, because your body-mind's energy is concentrated in your abdomen. Your overall energy is slow and needs to be permitted to be unimpeded as it focuses on turning nourishment into physical energy. After a meal, wait an hour before practice.

HOW OFTEN CAN I PRACTICE MUDRA?

You can practice as many mudras a day as you wish, but to obtain the full benefit that a mudra can give you, you will want to establish at least one three - minute set time during the day in which to grow comfortable with your mudra.

To feel the benefits faster, I recommend that you practice the mudra twice a day, each time for at least three minutes. Select a mudra that addresses a problem you have or a quality you want to develop, and make it a point to practice that mudra every day.

HOW LONG SHOULD I PRACTICE A MUDRA?

Your should practice a mudra in the beginning for at least three minutes a day, but when you have built up your strength and ability to hold the mudra and evoke its energy, you can extend your practice to eleven minutes. Ultimately, you may want to build up your practice to thirty-one minutes a day.

Most of the mudras will give you immediate results, in the form of more energy, clarity and peace of mind, or insight. More challenging or entrenched problems, however, will require more discipline and perseverance in your practice. It will take a few weeks of practice for the mudra to come into full effect and help you feel a profound transformation that will eliminate or resolve your problem.

MEDITATION

There are many different meditative techniques. If you have not meditated before, the simplest way to begin meditating is to find a quiet place and sit comfortably. Bring your attention to your breath: Exhale and inhale slowly through your nose and concentrate on your breath as it travels in and out of your body. As you concentrate, allow the awareness of your breath to still your mind and relax your body. You have begun to experience the essential state of meditation.

Meditation will lower your body temperature, so, when you plan to meditate for longer than eleven minutes, you should cover your back and shoulders with a shawl before sitting down. With mudras and proper breathing, you can achieve deeper levels of meditation. You will experience peace, relaxation, rejuvenation, and higher levels of consciousness.

Your intuition, patience, and wisdom will increase greatly, as will your personal magnetism and level of energetic vibration.

BREATHING

Proper breathing is essential when practicing a mudra. There are basically two types of breathing:

In LONG DEEP BREATHING, you take your time inhaling and exhaling slowly and completely, through your nose.

When you inhale, relax your abdomen and expand the chest.

When exhaling, deflate the chest and pull in the stomach to help expel the air. This technique of breathing will help you relax, calm down, and be more patient.

In the SHORT BREATH OF FIRE, inhale and exhale through the nose at a much faster pace. Focus on your navel point, expanding for inhalation and contracting on exhalation. Both parts are equal in time and can be quite rapid: two to three breaths per second.

This technique has a more invigorating effect.

Both techniques are very cleansing and healing.

During your mudra practice, it is best to use Long Deep Breathing except where noted.

CONCENTRATION

While practicing any mudra it is important to concentrate on the energy center of your Third Eye, which is between your eyebrows. Your Third Eye is the point of your body-mind that connects most easily to the higher sources of energy within you and around you.

As you practice meditation and mudra, if your mind wonders, gently bring your attention back to your breath and your mudra. Breathe in and out. You will experience a very powerful effect, a heightening of energy, throughout your entire body. Mudra practice affects each individual differently at different times. Sometimes you may feel a slight tingling sensation in your hands and arms; at other times, you may experience a sudden rush of energy through our spine. Allow yourself to feel and notice whatever comes up for you. Concentrating on the different feelings, allowing them to be there, will magnify the healing benefits to your body, mind and spirit.

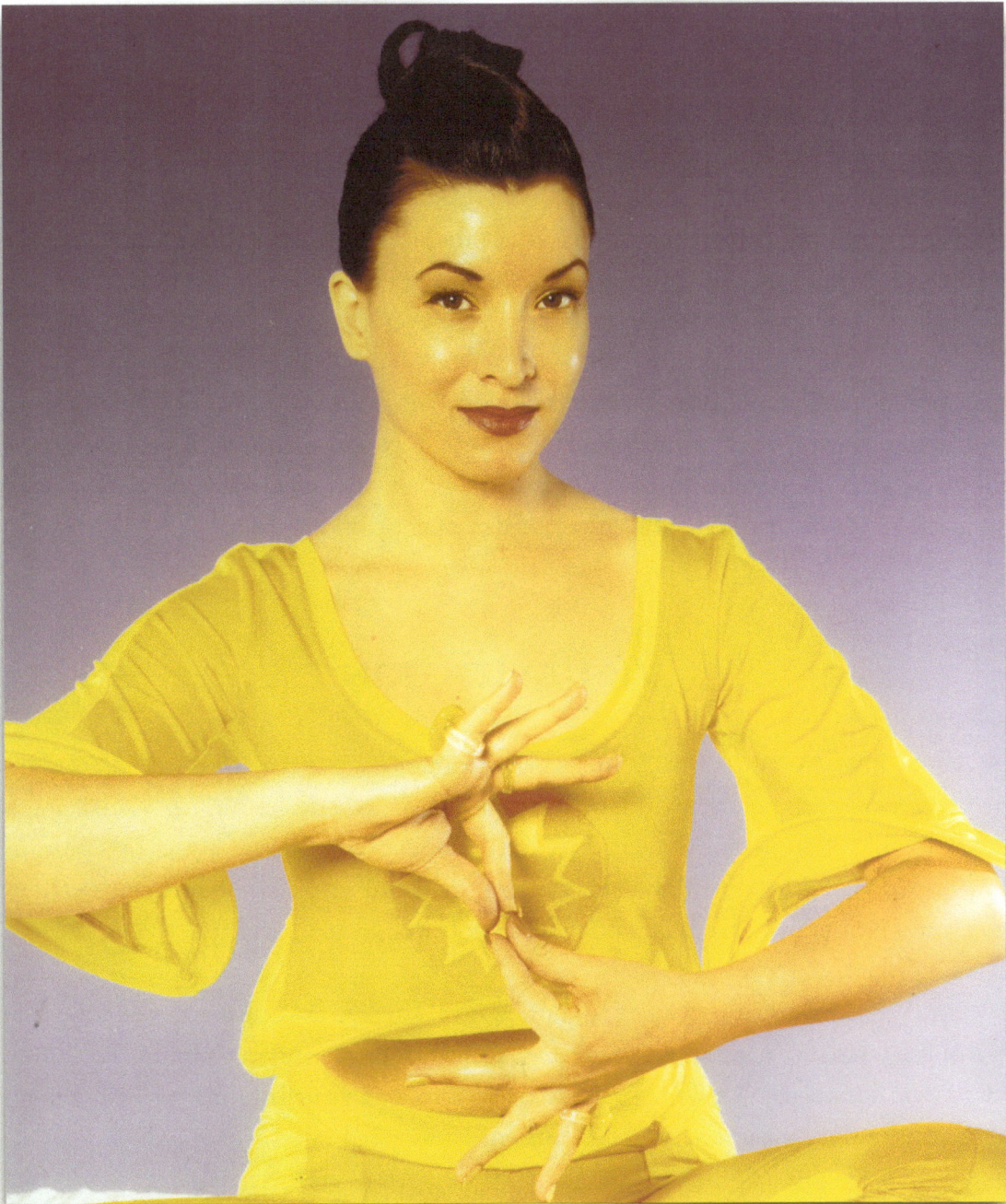

Your Third Eye center is the point between the eyebrows.
By focusing your mind's attention on this energy center of intuition,
you can practice visualization and receive guidance and visions.
It is your window to infinite possibilities.

Eye Movements

The eyes are an important element in the practice of mudra. How you use them will increase your concentration.

You can keep them half open and gently direct them to look over the tip of your nose. Do not cross your eyes to do this. Just look down and slightly in so that you perceive the end of your nose. This is a very beneficial exercise for your eyesight.

Another practice is to close your eyelids and gently aim your eyes upward toward the area of the Third Eye. If you need to keep your eyes open as you meditate, look into the middle distance and relax the eyelids. Most important, the eye focus should always be done *gently*. Never force your eyes into a painful or uncomfortable position.

Visualization

We all know how to daydream. Actually daydreaming is a form of visualization. In your mind you can create a picture, world, or dream in which you desire to live. Visualizing where you want to be and how you want to live and manifest your energy is the first step toward making your dream a reality. Mudra practice can help you actualize your dreams. The power of your mind is limitless. Live it, breathe it, and you will make it a reality.

For example: While practicing a mudra for anti aging, visualize in your mind a healthy, youthful glow around your face. See yourself and your face vibrant and recharged. By adding the power of your mind to your daily practice of mudra and visualization, you will change and improve your outlook, your energy, and your entire life.

As another example, when practicing a mudra for insight, see yourself as having reached a happy solution for a problem you've been trying to resolve. Visualize how you would feel if your concern were over. From this visualization will emerge a positive approach to creating a good outcome.

Positive Affirmations and Prayer

When you meditate, your mind becomes fine-tuned to your body's needs and you gain in healing capacity. It is important before you meditate to make a positive affirmation for yourself. You can also affirm positive energy for another person, just as you would in a prayer.

Example: When practicing the mudra for dieting it is beneficial to affirm:
"I am eating only healthful food. I am healthy, trim, and full. I am sticking to my diet."
This simple affirmation will have a positive effect on you.

When meditating or praying for someone else, it is helpful to see them surrounded by white or violet light and affirm: "My friend is healthy, happy, full of life, and smiling."
Your affirmation should always be formed in the resent tense. "I am calm," not "I will be or want to be calm." or, "I see the solution in my meditation." This positive statement creates powerful energy vibrations. Your energy is sent out into the Universe and manifests your desires and intentions, enabling you to accomplish your goals successfully, honorably, and compassionately. Prayer and affirmations are especially powerful during the practice of mudra when your mind is calm and your concentration is magnified.

Mantra

While you may prefer to practice your mudra and meditation using your affirmation, you may also want to try using a mantra. Mantras are ancient Sanskrit healing words that have a powerful effect on your entire being when chanted repeatedly during meditation or mudra practice. The hard palate in your mouth has fifty-eight energy points that connect to your entire body. Stimulating these points with sound vibrations affects your mental and physical energy. Certain sounds that stimulate these points have a very healing quality. When you repeat aloud or whisper these ancient mantras or scientific healing-sound combinations, the meridians on your hard palate are activated in a specific order that re-patterns the energy of your whole system. There are three basic mantras that you will find in this book in different combinations:

EK ONG KAR
One Creator, God Is One

SA TA NA MA
Infinity, Birth, Death, Rebirth

HAR HARE HAREE
WAHE GURU
Hah-rah; hah-ray; hah-ree; wa -hay; guh-roo
God is the Creator of Supreme Power and Wisdom

Not every mudra practice requires a mantra. All mudras can be practiced in silence to the rhythm of your breathing. You can use the mantras when you are struggling with a restless mind, since focusing on the words will help center you. Follow your intuition during the mudra practice and if you are drawn to chanting the mantras, try them when you feel it is right. You will experience profound peace, joy, and passion. Your soul will sing with the Universe.

THE MANTRA PRONUNCIATION GUIDE

A like *a* in about
AA like the *a* in want
AY like *ay* in say
AI like the *a* in sand
I like the *i* in bit
U like the *u* in put
OO like the *oo* in good
O like the *o* in no
E like the *ay* in say
EE like the *e* in meet
AAU like the *ow* in now
SAT rhymes with "what"
NAM rhymes with "mom"
WAHE – sounds like wa-hay
GU – sounds like "put"
Emphasize the"ch" at the end of every " such."Pronounce the consonant v softly.
Roll the *rs* slightly. When chanting the mantra like " Haree Har Haree Har,"
make sure you do not move your lips, and pronounce it with the tongue only.

THE HANDS

Both hands and all ten fingers have individual, distinct meanings. Each corresponds to the energy of a different body part and to the energy of our solar system. The right hand is influenced by the Sun and represents the male side of one's nature. The left hand is ruled by the Moon and represents the female aspect of one's nature.

The right hand is the receiver while the left is the giver of positive powers. These meanings are also reflected in the hand positions of mudras.
Each finger is associated with a special ability, tendency, or characteristic and how it affects your life.

The **THUMB** symbolizes God. When the rest of your fingers connect to the thumb you symbolically bow to God. The Thumb is associated with the planet Mars and represents willpower, logic, love, and ego. The angle it makes with the rest of your hand when relaxed indicates your character. A distance between the thumb and index fingers of around ninety degrees indicates you are generous, kindhearted, and giving. A distance of about sixty degrees suggests a logical, rational character. A thirty-degree space indicates a secretive, sensitive, and cautious person. A long, strong thumb reveals a strong personality, willpower, and the ability to change your destiny.

The **INDEX** finger is influenced by the planet Jupiter and represents your knowledge, wisdom, sense of power, and self-confidence.

The **MIDDLE** finger is the indicator of the planet Saturn and relates to patience and emotional control. Therefore, it has a balancing effect on your life.

The **RING** finger connects with the Sun and represents vitality, life energy, and your health. It corresponds to your sense of family and matters of the heart.

The **LITTLE** finger is the indicator for the planet Mercury, which rules your ability to communicate, be creative, appreciate beauty, and achieve inner calm.

The tips of fingers can reveal qualities of different natures.
An oval fingertip can signify an impulsive person who needs motivation. A pointy fingertip is common for an independent, active person, and a square fingertip shows a logical and practical person.

THE CHAKRAS

Within our body, we have seven major nerve and energy centers that are located along the spine. The first is at the base of spine, the seventh at the top of the head. These centers are called Chakras. Their energy is always spinning clockwise within our bodies and influences - and is influenced by – our emotional, spiritual, and physical health. In order to feel balanced and in harmony within ourselves and our environments, it is important that we know about these centers and their functions.

FIRST CHAKRA
Represents: Survival, food, shelter, courage, will, foundation
Location: Base of spine
Gland: Gonads
Color: Red

SECOND CHAKRA
Represents: Sex, creativity, procreation, family, inspiration
Location: Sex organs
Gland: Adrenal
Color: Orange

THIRD CHAKRA
Represents: Ego, emotional center, the intellect, the mind
Location: Solar plexus
Gland: Pancreas
Color: Yellow

FOURTH CHAKRA
Represents: Unconditional true love, devotion, faith, compassion
Location: Heart region
Gland: Thymus
Color: Green or pink

FIFTH CHAKRA
Represents: Voice, truth, communication, higher knowledge
Location: Throat
Gland: Thyroid
Color: Blue

SIXTH CHAKRA

Represents: Third Eye, vision, intuition
Location: Third Eye
Gland: Pineal
Color: Indigo

SEVENTH CHAKRA

Represents: Universal God consciousness, the heavens, unity, humility
Location: Top of the head, crown
Gland: Pituitary
Color: Violet

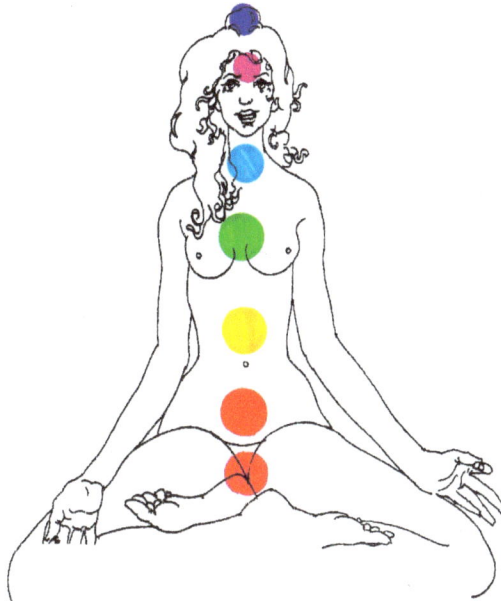

CHAKRAS IN THE BODY

Base Chakra: Foundation
Second Chakra: Sexuality
Third Chakra: Ego
Fourth Chakra: Love
Fifth Chakra: Truth
Sixth Chakra: Intuition
Seventh Chakra: Divine Wisdom

Mudras are a powerful tool for energizing and balancing each Chakra, activating the electric current in our body, and releasing the limitless power from within. Example: When practicing the mudra for divine worship, you can visualize healing Chakra colors surrounding, filling, and energizing your body, starting with the First Chakra and continuing up to your head, the Crown Chakra.

ELECTRIC CURRENTS

Besides the seven Chakras within our body, there are seventy-two thousand electric currents or channels called *Nadis* - pronounced "nah-dees". They run from all different body points, from the tips of the toes to the top of the head. The Nadis also affect your entire system. Keeping these energy currents activated and full of powerful flowing energy is essential to your wellbeing. Each mudra redirects, activates, and empowers the energy flowing through those channels, and stimulates the brain centers, nerves, and organs, with benefits to your entire neuromuscular, physical, and glandular system.

HEALING COLORS

Using the healing power of colors can also enhance your mudra practice. The rainbow colors of the Chakras heal and reenergize corresponding body parts. You can surround yourself with appropriate colors whenever you meditate or visualize the colors as you practice mudras.

For instance, when practicing the mudra for powerful insight, you can visualize yourself surrounded by white or violet light. This will enhance your intuitive capacity. Wearing a certain color will also influence your entire outlook on life.

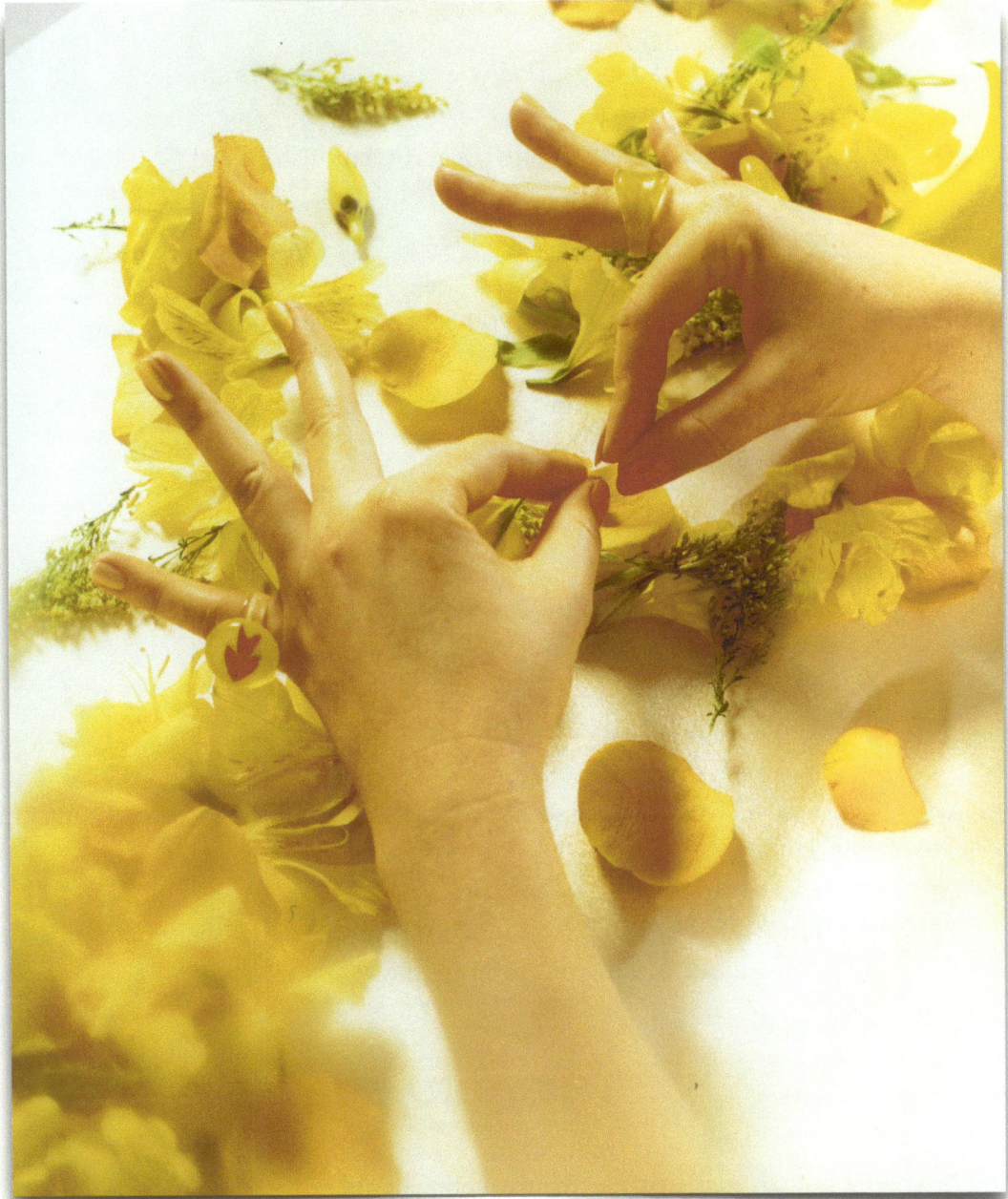

MUDRA OF YIN - FEMININE POWER

Examples:

RED will positively affect your vitality, ground you, and connect you to the earth.

ORANGE will empower your sexuality, creativity, and relationships.

YELLOW makes you feel energized and full of fire.

GREEN is good for the days when you need to heal your heart and feel love.

BLUE has a calming, peaceful effect on your aura or the energy field surrounding your body, and will help you see and speak the truth.

INDIGO will enhance your intuition and sixth sense.

VIOLET is a great centering and calming color that will help you connect with the universal healing powers.

BLACK will help you communicate as the leader.

WHITE will make you feel cleansed and pure, and will help clear you of any negative feelings or depression.

Reflect on the messages your body sends you every morning, and see what color you feel most drawn to and comfortable wearing on different days.

THE AURA

Our aura or energy body is made of electromagnetic energy vibrations that include color, light, sound, heat, and emotions. It surrounds us as a glow that is usually invisible. With practice and concentration, however, you can learn to see auras. The mudra for feeling the energy body is particularly effective in helping you discern auras. When our invisible magnetic force is very vibrant, it signifies good health, personal power, and a healing capacity.

Useful Mudra Tips

Some mudras may seem at first to be very similar to each other. Yet each is, in practice quite different: every detail in the posture of your hands and fingers is important and significant. When you pay close attention to your practice of mudras, you will feel the difference. As we discussed, every fingertip is connected to a different body center and energy current. Concentrate on the mudra as you practice, and notice the different feeling and effect that each brings to you. You can practice one specific mudra at a time or combine a few in one sitting. Listen to your body.

Example: If you are stressed out and need to concentrate, practice the mudra for preventing stress. After three minutes, go on to the mudra for concentration. As you try different combinations, your body-mind's logic and intuition will guide you. That is the beauty of the mudras — you can practice them anyplace, anytime, in whatever order you desire. This ancient science of the mudra is complex in benefits, yet simple in practice.

Now that you have some background about the power and history of mudras, and some rudiments of meditation practice, you're ready to begin trying some mudras and applying their energy to your life. In the next sections, you will find mudras for your soul, mudras for healing physical conditions, and mudras for easing troublesome states of mind, among others. Every one of these fifty-two traditional mudras can be a spiritual tool for you and help you in your own process of self-discovery and creative problem solving. I hope that they will enable you to find more insight, pleasure, and power on your life journey.

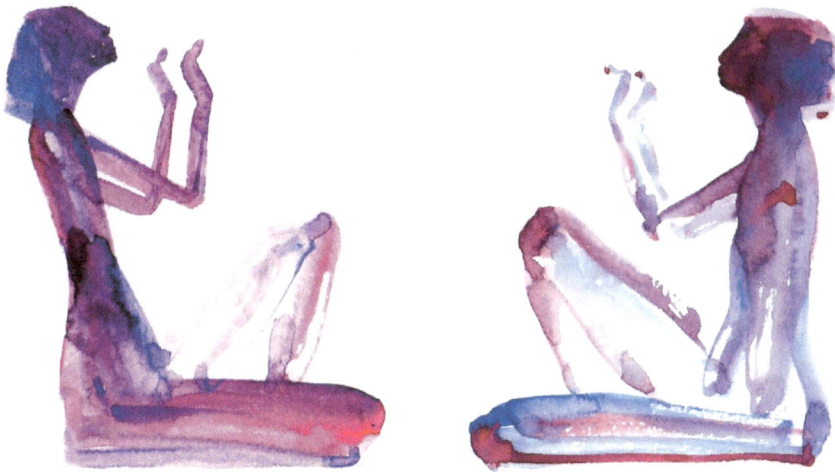

MUDRAS

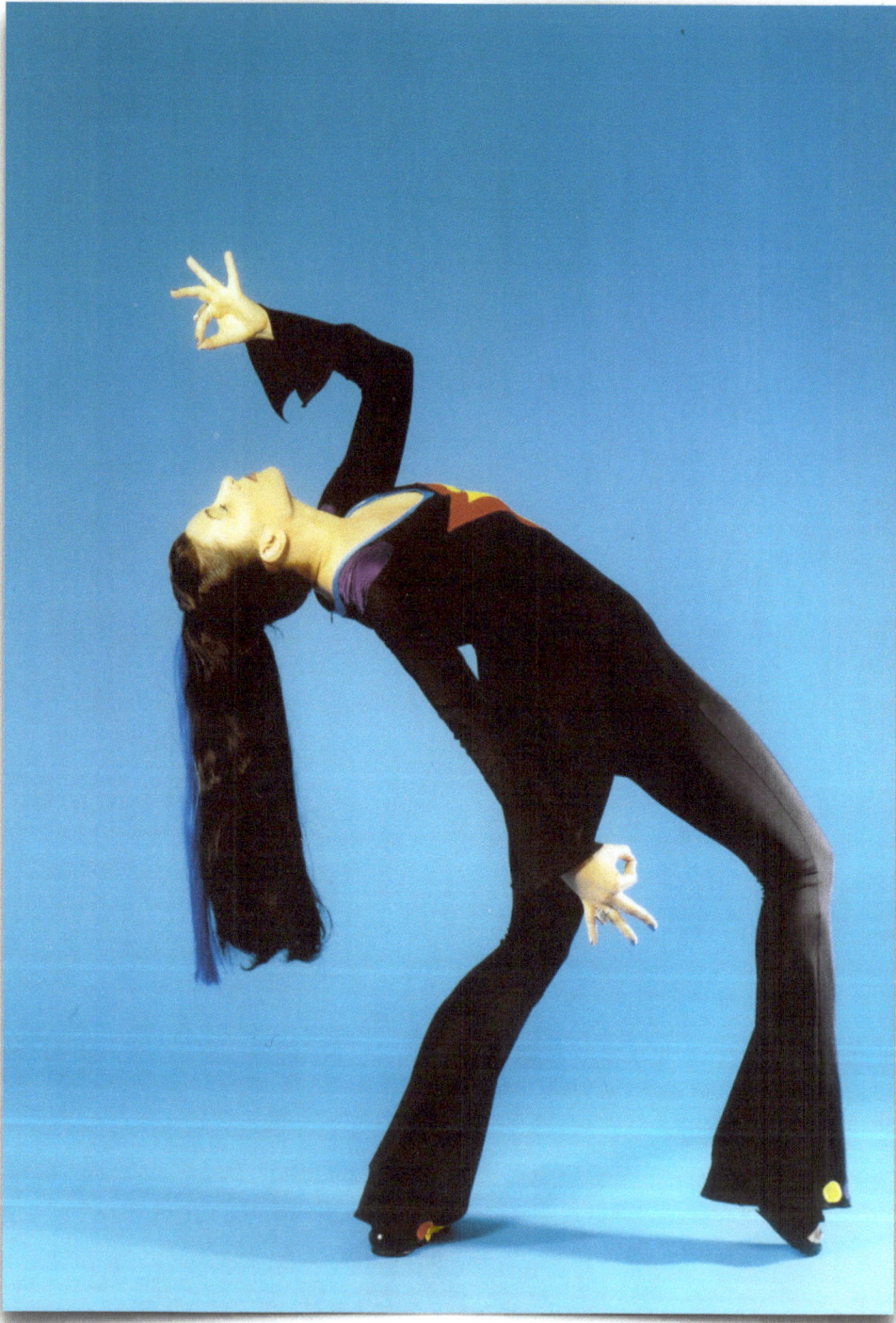

MUDRAS
FOR YOUR SOUL

YOUR SOUL IS IMMORTAL...
WORSHIP IT.

This chapter contains sixteen mudras that will help you trust and connect with the energy of divine love, power, and wisdom, which is the source and sustainer of all living beings. When you need guidance, love, and inner strength, you can nourish your soul with the practice of mudra. Once you have met your own needs, you can continue to build up your own energy so that you are empowered and connected to the Universe, able to help others in need.

You may practice one mudra a day or several. These will help you feel filled with peace, joy, and the knowledge that you are deeply loved and protected by your creator.
After the practice, take a few moments in complete peace and silence to feel the effects. If you do your part, holding yourself open to the Divine, the rest will be done for you.

MUDRA FOR DIVINE WORSHIP

The essential goal of yoga is to become centered, calm, and at one with the Divine, God, or the Universal intelligence. Being respectful of the Higher Power, relying on it and being in tune with the Universe, are prerequisites for inner peace. When we realize we are all created equal, and all connected with the ultimate source of spiritual energy, we feel empowered and in harmony.

The Mudra for Divine Worship is the universal symbol for prayer and has been used worldwide by saints and sages of many cultures and spiritual traditions. It sometimes begins with a bow to show our humility before the Divine Power. Connecting the palm and all fingertips symbolizes the unity and oneness with the Divine and magnifies the healing energy within.

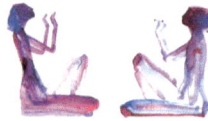

CHAKRA: All Chakras

COLOR: All Colors

MANTRA: EK ONG KAR
~ One Creator, God is One ~
Repeat mentally with each breath

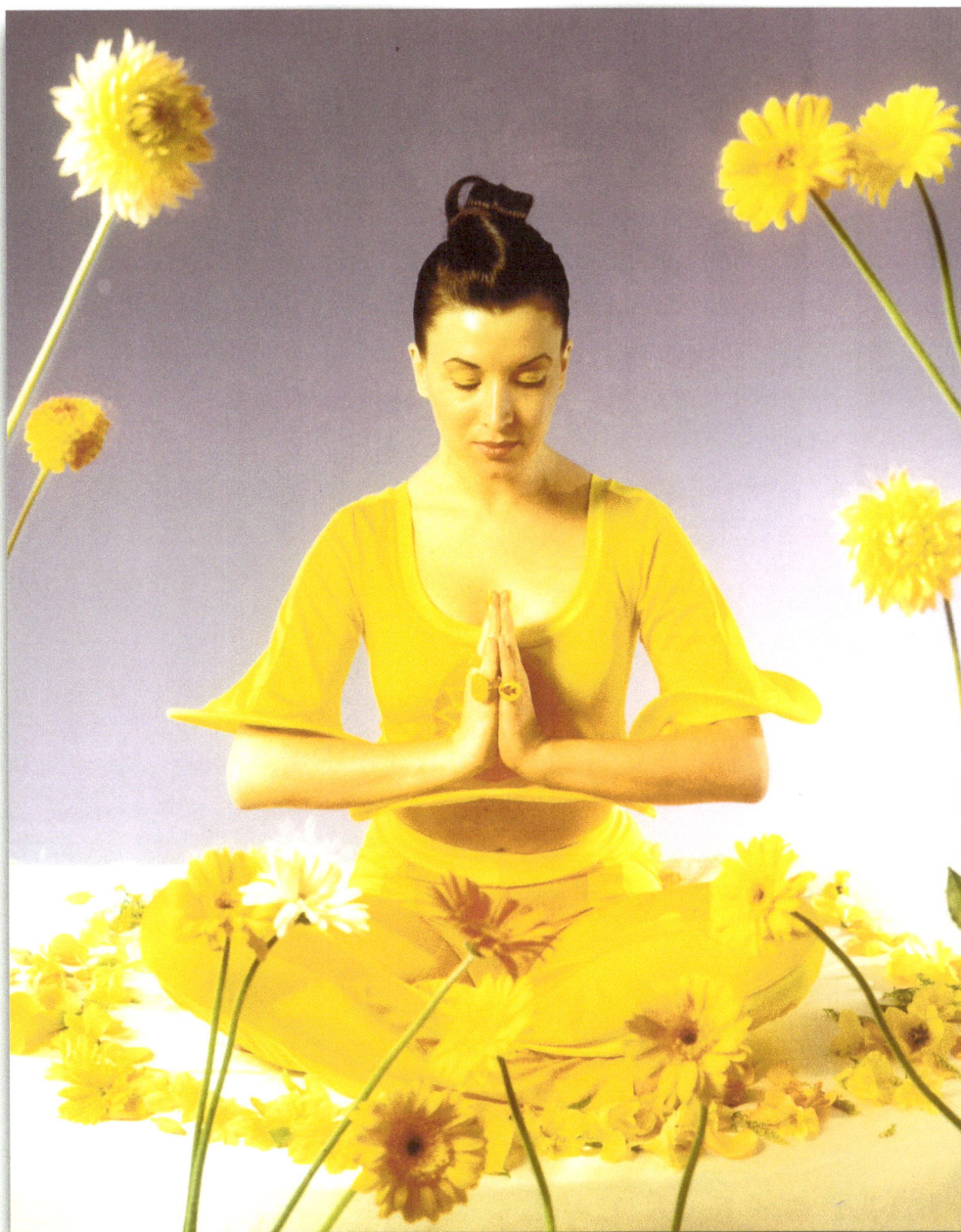

Sit in a comfortable position. Place your palms together in front of your chest. Concentrate on the Third Eye center.

BREATH: LONG AND DEEP.

Relax your mind and continue for at least three minutes.

MUDRA FOR HAPPINESS

Happiness is a state of mind that comes from within, just as true beauty emanates from our internal spiritual state. You can choose to make a conscious effort to greet each day and its events with a happy, positive outlook and to appreciate what you have. With regular practice of this mudra, you can be happy, look happy, and be a positive example to others. Make is a point to be happy today, tomorrow, and for the rest of your life.

The power of this mudra has a great effect
on your state of mind and helps you feel joyful.

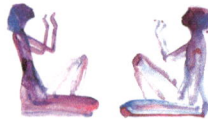

CHAKRA: Heart – 4

COLOR: Green

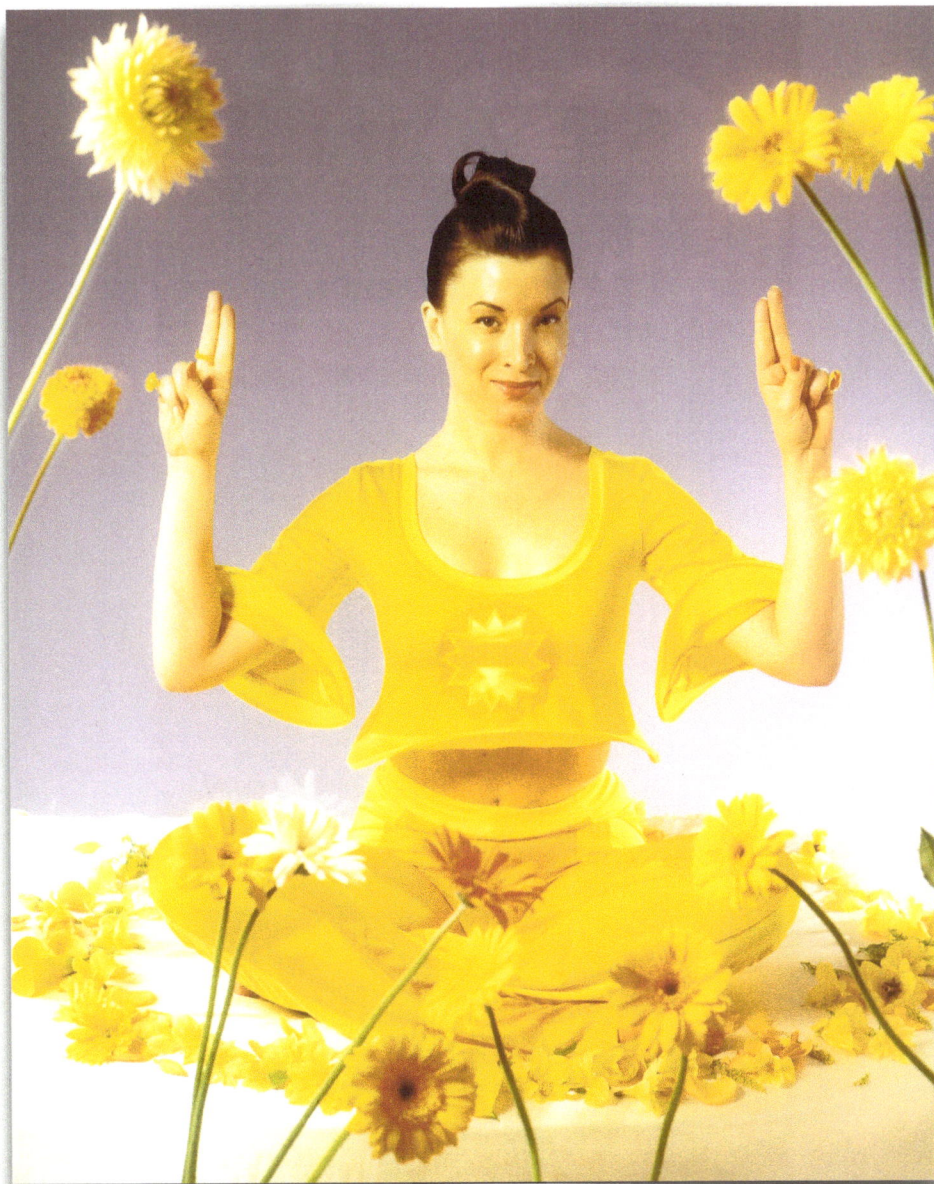

Sit comfortably with a straight spine. Curl the ring and small fingers and press them into your palms firmly but gently with the thumbs. Keep the first two fingers pointing straight up. Keep your spine straight and lift the elbows to the side and away from the body.

BREATH: CONTROLLED, LONG AND DEEP, CONCENTRATING ON THE THIRD EYE AS YOU BREATHE.

MUDRA FOR LOVE

Whether it is love for a child, spouse, parent, friend, lover, or any other living creature, love transforms us. It makes life worth living. Sharing our love with the world and teaching others about love is the spiritual mission at the base of every individual's life. Love yourself, humankind, and God, and you will achieve any goal.

This mudra activates the energy currents
that stimulate the emotion of love.

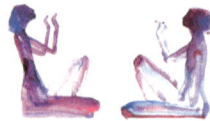

CHAKRA: Heart – 4

COLOR: Green

MANTRA: SAT NAM WAHE GURU
~ God Is Truth, His is The Supreme Power and Wisdom ~
Eight counts of breathing in, exhale to one count.
Mentally repeat the mantra twice when you inhale

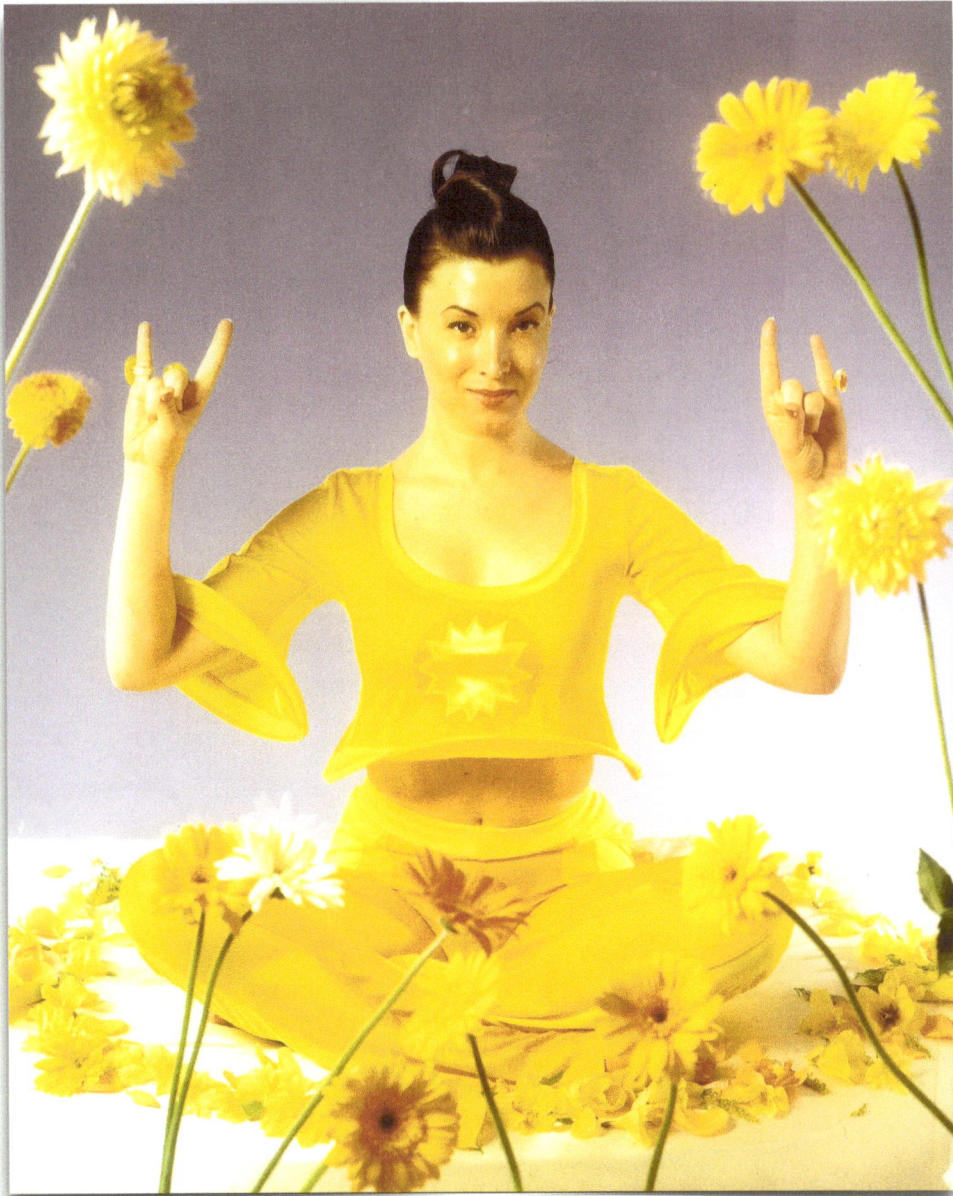

Sit with a straight spine. Curl the middle and ring fingers down into your palms while extending the thumbs and other fingers. Keep your elbows up, concentrate, and continue for a few minutes, feel love and light around you.

BREATH: EIGHT COUNTS INHALATION, ONE STRONG EXHALATION.

MUDRA FOR UNIVERSAL ENERGY AND ETERNITY

We use only a small portion of our conscious mind ever day. The practice of this mudra will stimulate your entire brain so that you can expand its capacity. By keeping energy flowing throughout your body and mind, and by learning how to recharge them every day, you stay in closer connection to the energy of life and the Universe as a whole.

This mudra is beneficial for your whole system.
The hands are your channels to draw the life energy
into your body, mind, and soul.

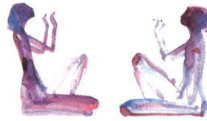

CHAKRA: Base of Spine –1
Crown – 7

COLOR: Red, Violet

MANTRA: HAR HARE HAREE WAHE GURU
~ God the Creator of Supreme Power and Wisdom,
the Spiritual Teacher and Guide Through Darkness ~
Repeat mentally with each breath

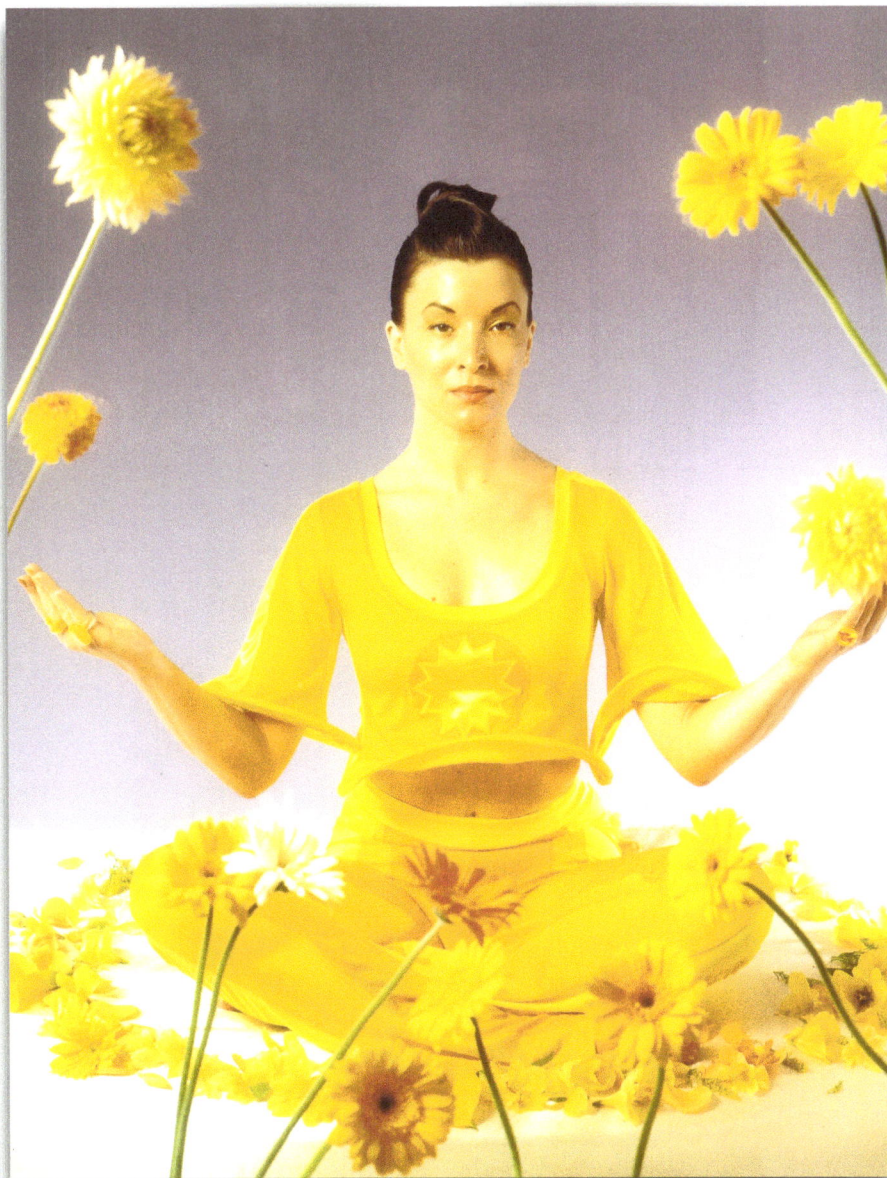

Sit with a straight spine. Bend your elbows, open your arms out to either side, and raise your hands up to heart level. Your arms and torso will form two V's. Keep palms facing up toward the sky with fingers close together. Concentrate on your Third Eye and feel the flow of energy into your palms. Relax and feel a deep sense of peace.

BREATH: LONG, DEEP, AND CONTROLLED.

MUDRA FOR TRUST

No relationship can exist for any length of time without trust. But first you must have faith and trust in yourself, your spirit, and in the greater wisdom of the Universe. Do you trust yourself? Do you have faith in yourself? We are all connected to the ultimate creative force and Divine Spirit, which surround us and also lie within us. We are never alone and we are never forgotten. Self-trust and spiritual trust will help you attract people and relationships in which you have faith. The power of victory is always within you. It all starts with you.

This mudra will help you build trust, faith, and spiritual balance
so that you can stand up to any challenge and
see God in every aspect of your life.

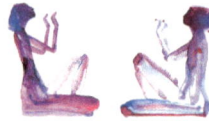

CHAKRA: Crown – 7

COLOR: Violet

MANTRA: HAR HAR HAR WAHE GURU
~ God's Creation, his Supreme power and Wisdom ~
Repeat mentally with each breath

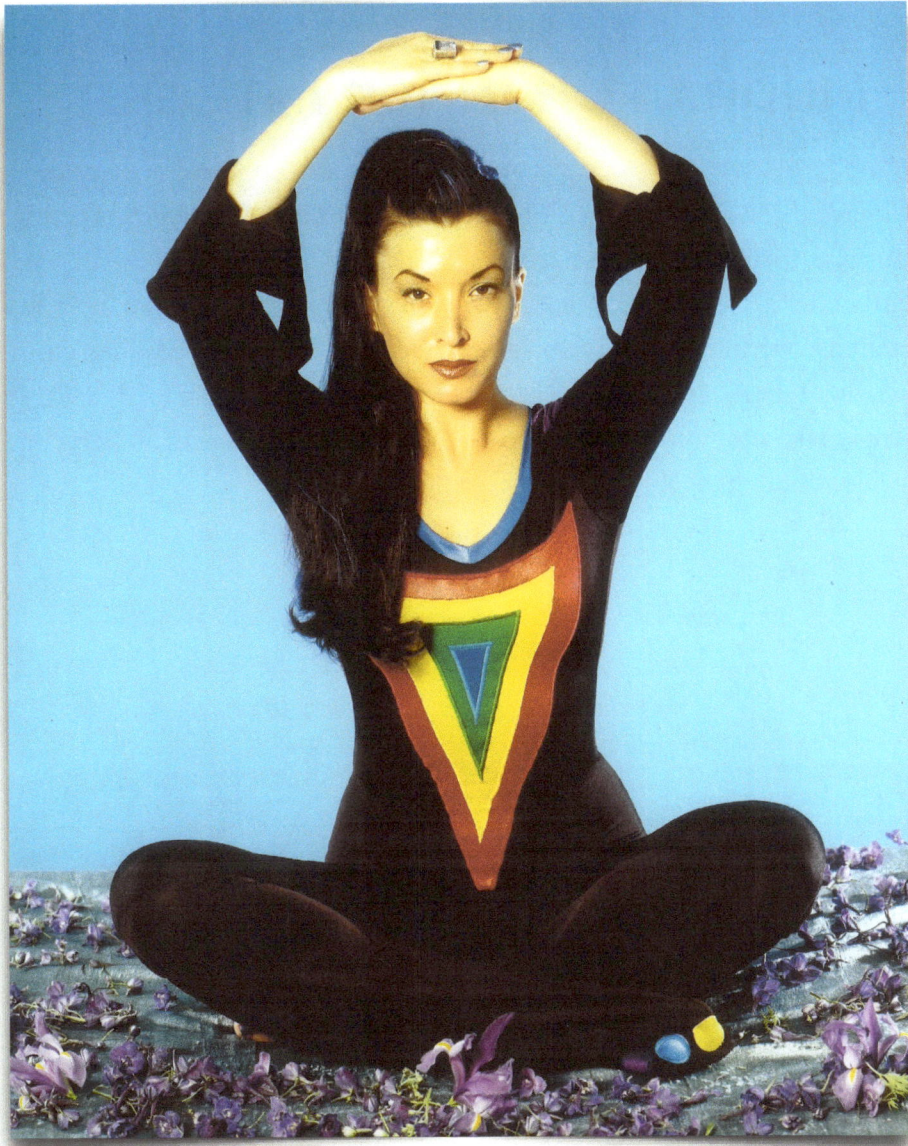

Sit with a straight back and make a circle with your arms arched up over your head, palms down. Women should put their right palm on top of the left. Men put the left palm on top of the right. Lightly press the thumb tips together, keep your back straight, and visualize a protective circle of energy all around you.

BREATH: SHORT, FAST BREATH OF FIRE, FOCUSING ON THE NAVEL. Hold the mudra and continue for a few minutes. Then relax and sit still.

Mudra for Inner Integrity

We all encounter difficult situations that test our character. Even when we feel the impulse to react emotionally to a particular challenge, however, we must remember to act in accordance with most intelligent, rational response. In maintaining our integrity we can save ourselves and our loved ones from a lot of sorrow, regret, and unnecessary pain. When you are faced with such a challenge, take a few minutes to be by yourself, practice this powerful mudra, and notice your change of heart and mind.

This mudra will strengthen your ability to keep your presence of mind and inner integrity so that you can make correct choices and responses under stress.

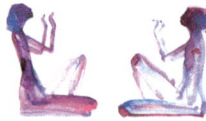

CHAKRA: Throat – 5
Third Eye – 6

COLOR: Blue, Indigo

MANTRA: SAT NAM
~ Truth Is God's Name, One in Spirit ~
Repeat mentally with each breath

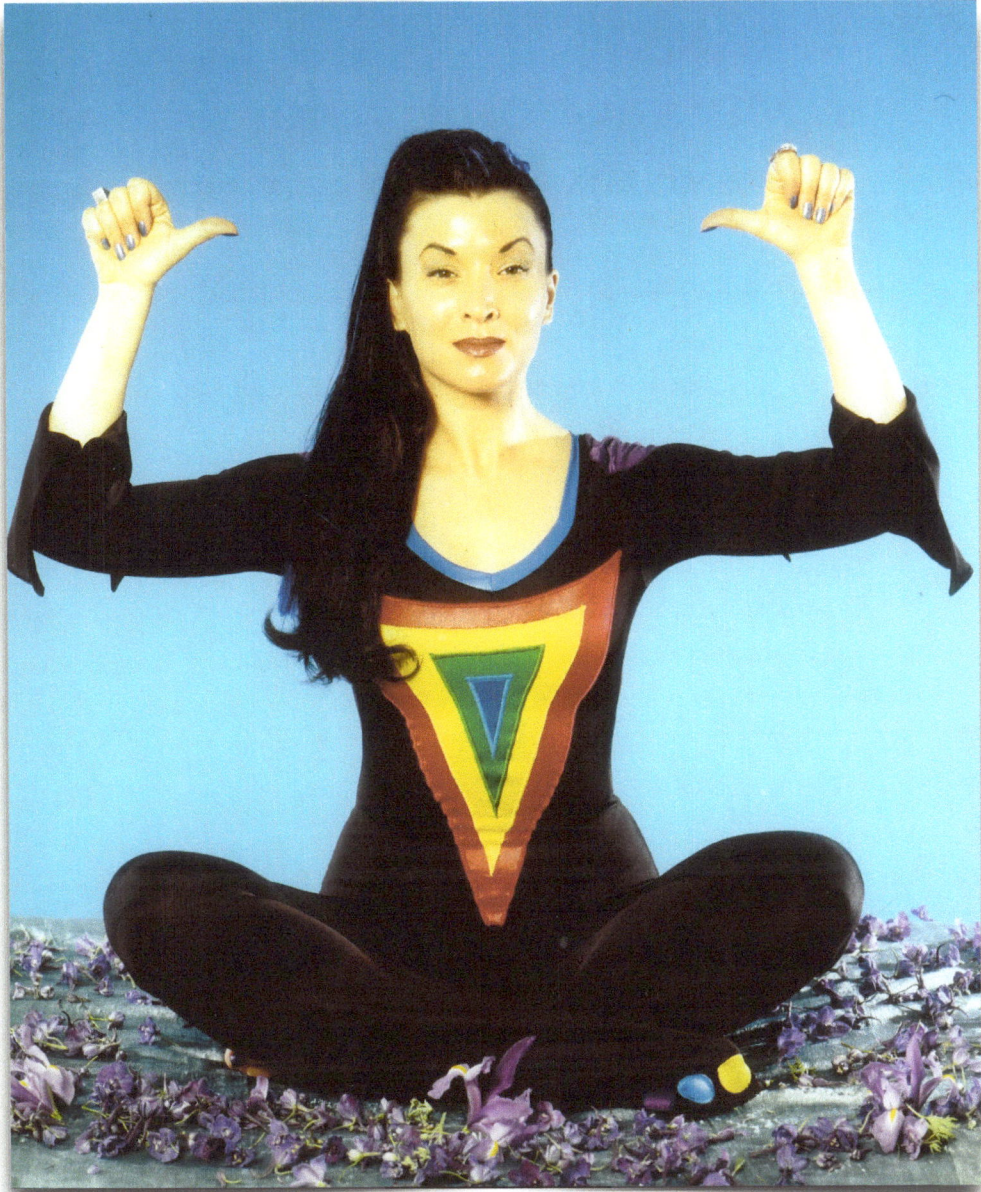

Sit with a straight spine, your upper arms raised parallel to the ground, your elbows bent so your forearms are perpendicular. Bring your hands to ear level, palms out. Curl your fingers inward so that they touch the palms. Extend your thumbs straight out and point them toward your temples. Practice for at least three minutes, then relax.

BREATH: SHORT, FAST BREATH OF FIRE, FOCUSING ON THE NAVEL.

MUDRA FOR EVOKING INNER STRENGTH

We all possess great reserves of inner power and wisdom. Within this innate understanding are all the answers to our problems. The practice of this mudra will help you tap into that well of inner strength. The mudra puts you in touch with the universal, everlasting force that lies within you.

As you hold the hand formations in front of your chest,
you are activating the power centers of the Third and Fourth Chakras,
which will give you inner strength and courage.

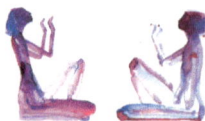

CHAKRA: Solar plexus – 3
Heart – 4

COLOR: Yellow, Green

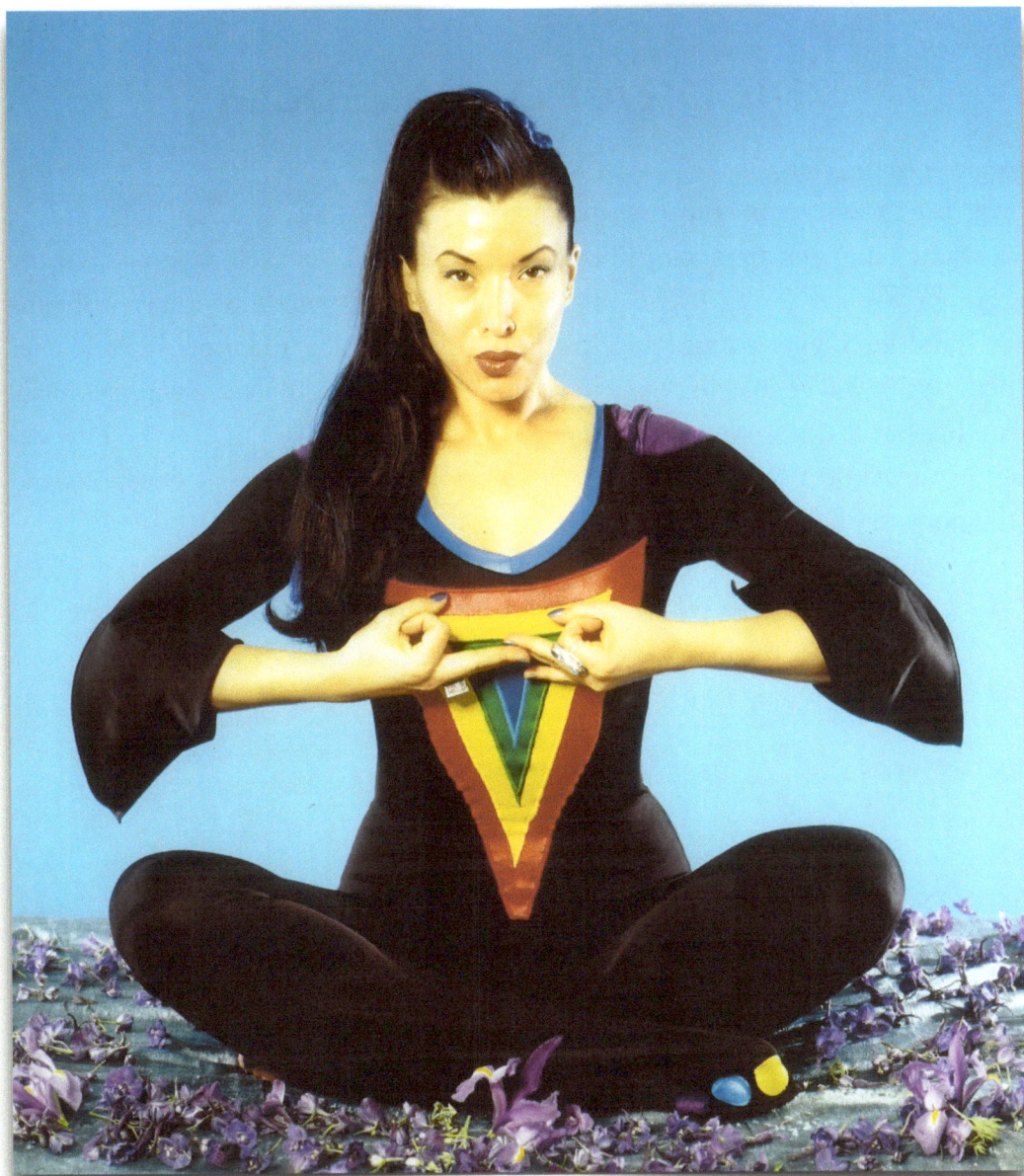

Sit with a straight spine. Curl your index fingers and curl your thumbs over them. Straighten the other three fingers. Your right hand is slightly under the left hand. Place your hands in front of your chest, keeping your elbows up out to the sides so that your forearms and hands make lines parallel to the ground.
BREATH: INHALE IN FOUR STROKES THROUGH THE NOSE, SHAPE YOUR LIPS INTO AN O, EXHALE WITH A WHISTLE. Continue for three minutes, then relax and feel the power within you.

MUDRA FOR WISDOM

We can connect to our innate, divine wisdom by clearing our minds, concentrating, and practicing this ancient mudra. It will help you resolve any conflict you are facing by helping you see beyond your individual problems and into the bigger picture and higher meaning of any situation. This greater perspective will enable you to help yourself and others. This is a very powerful mudra, but it does require devoted practice. Do it every day for three weeks and you will be able to perceive more easily the answers to your questions and the purposes behind your life's challenges.

This mudra stimulates the mind nerve and clears your
access to higher knowledge and wisdom.

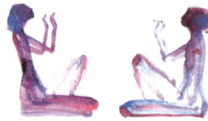

CHAKRA: Third Eye – 6

COLOR: Indigo

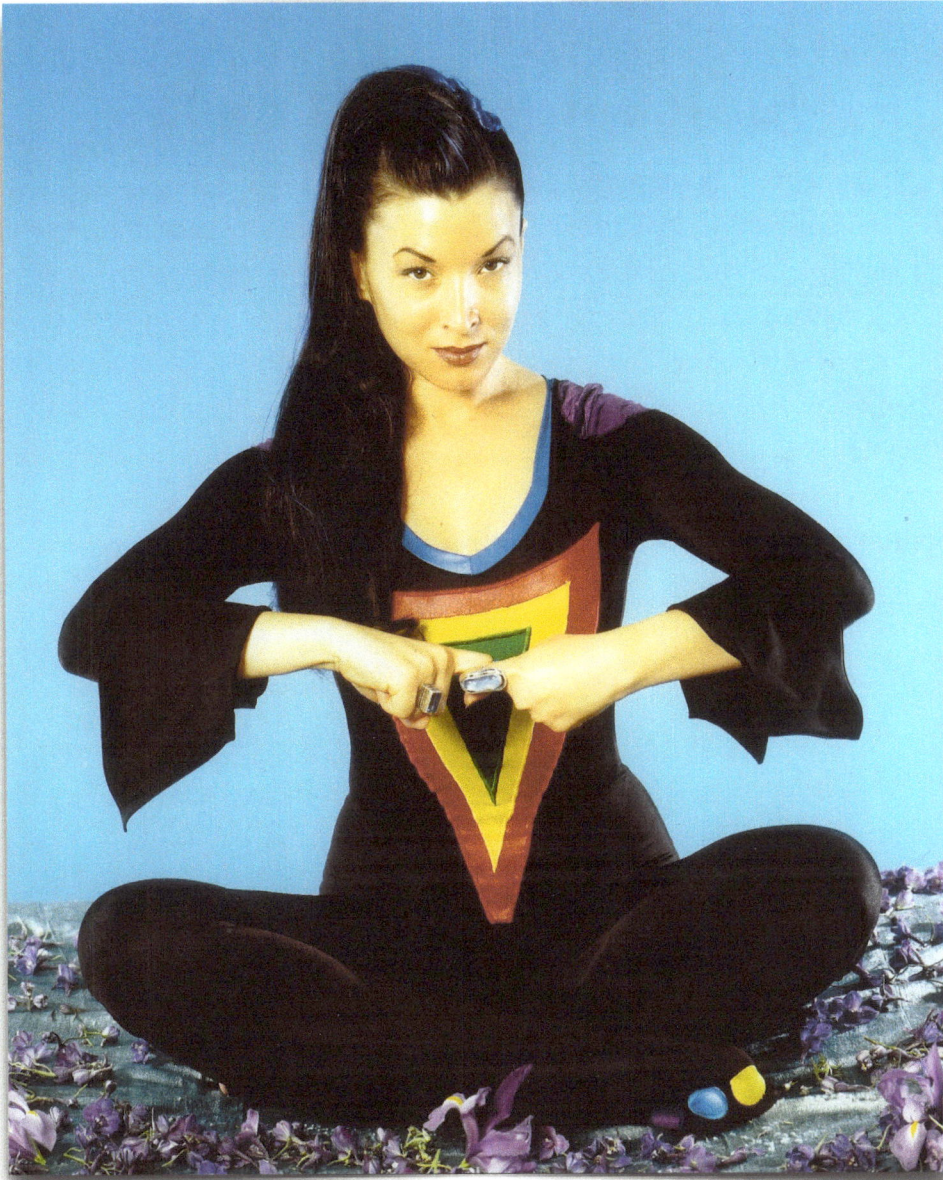

Sit with a straight back. Curl your thumbs into your palms and your last three fingers over them. Leaving your index fingers extended. Keep your shoulders down and relaxed, and raise your elbows out to either side. Bring your curled hands in front of your chest and hook the index fingers together, right palm facing the ground, left palm facing your chest, forearms parallel to the floor.

BREATHE: LONG, DEEP AND SLOW.

Hold the mudra for three to eleven minutes, relax, and sit still.

MUDRA FOR GENTLENESS

There are times when we are simply in a bad space at a bad time and feel harsh and unkind toward those closest to us. We may react unthinkingly, and while we may not mean what we say or do, our words or behavior can be very damaging. If we never learned or experienced calmness and gentleness as children, it may be difficult for us to be kind as adults. Gentleness is one of the highest soul qualities, however, and by cultivating it, we will be able to attract kind and loving people into our lives, and achieve a greater level of happiness and fulfillment.

This mudra will adjust the electromagnetic field of the brain and bring you calm and gentleness.

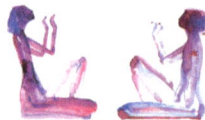

CHAKRA: Throat – 5
Crown – 7
COLOR: Blue, Violet
MANTRA: HARI ONG HARI ONG TAT SAT
~ God in Action, the Ultimate Truth ~
Repeat mentally with each breath

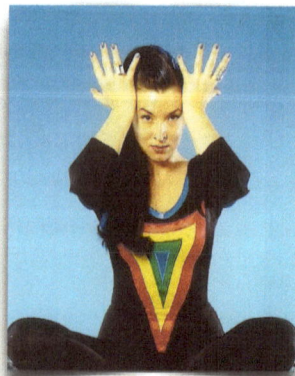

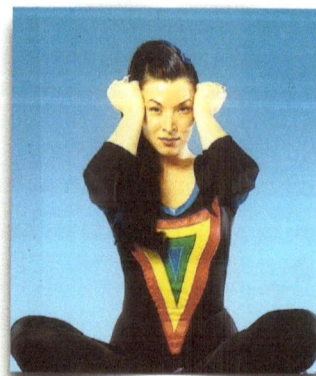

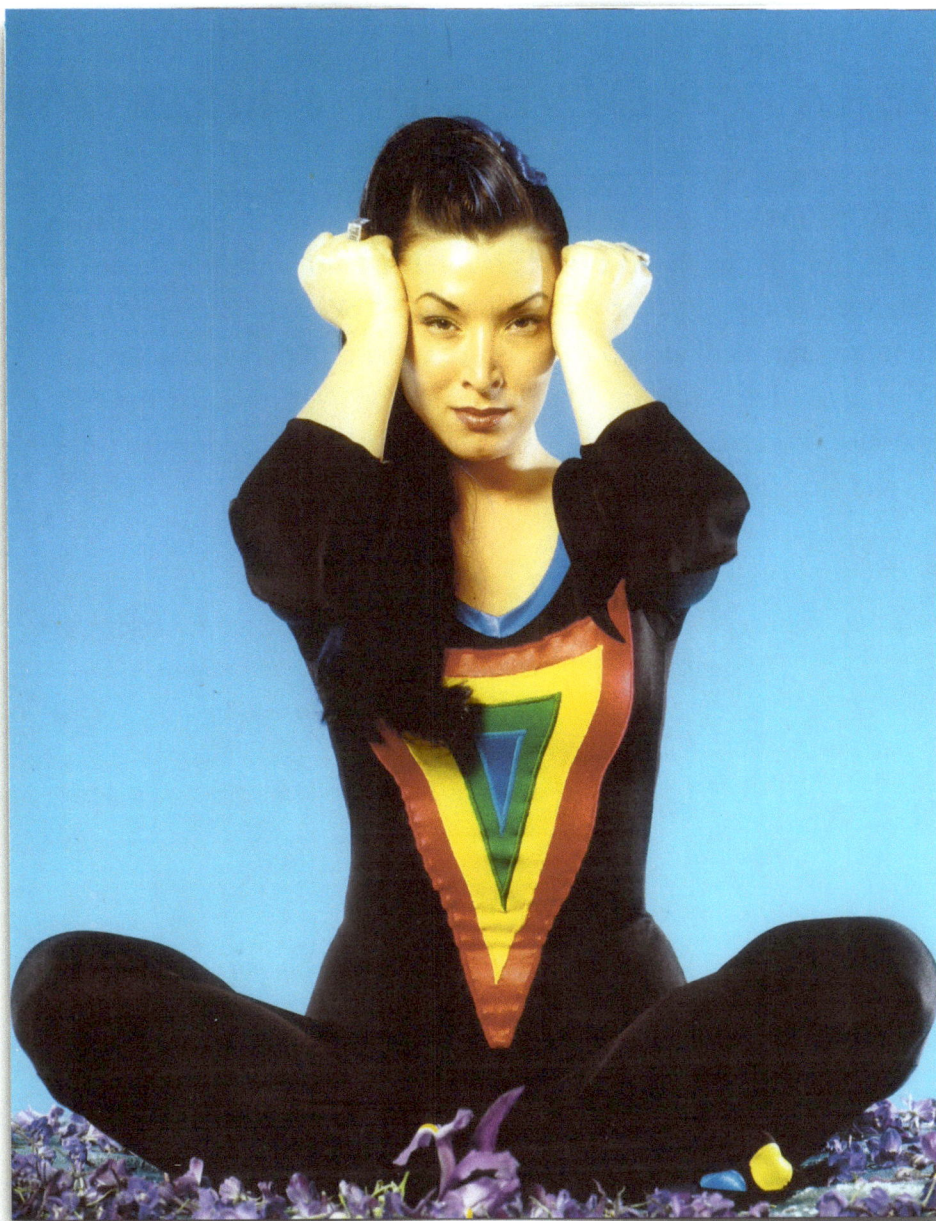

Sit with a straight back. Make fists and bring the outer (thumb) side of each fist to either side of your temples. Press the fists slightly against the temples and place the fingers apart. Close your eyes. Then make fists again, keeping the thumb sides pressing against the temples.

BREATH: LONG, DEEP AND SLOW.

Practice for a few minutes, relax, and sit still.

MUDRA FOR DEVELOPING MEDITATION

Some of us may struggle at the thought of sitting still for more than a few seconds. All of us have trouble sitting at different points in our life. Meditation is only a matter of discipline and practice. Learning how to still your mind and meditate even for three-minute period is essential for your well-being. A short daily meditation will change your life for the better, and the sooner you start the sooner you will experience wonderful results on all levels and areas of your life.

This is a meditation for someone who cannot meditate.
It will bring one-pointedness and serenity to the most outrageous or scattered mind.
The mantra will help you focus with the one universal force,
"the heartbeat of life," that lies within us all.

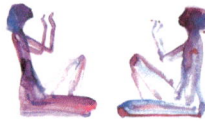

CHAKRA: All Chakras
COLOR: All Colors

MANTRA: SAT NAM
~ Truth Is God's Name, One in Spirit ~
Repeat mentally with each beat of your pulse

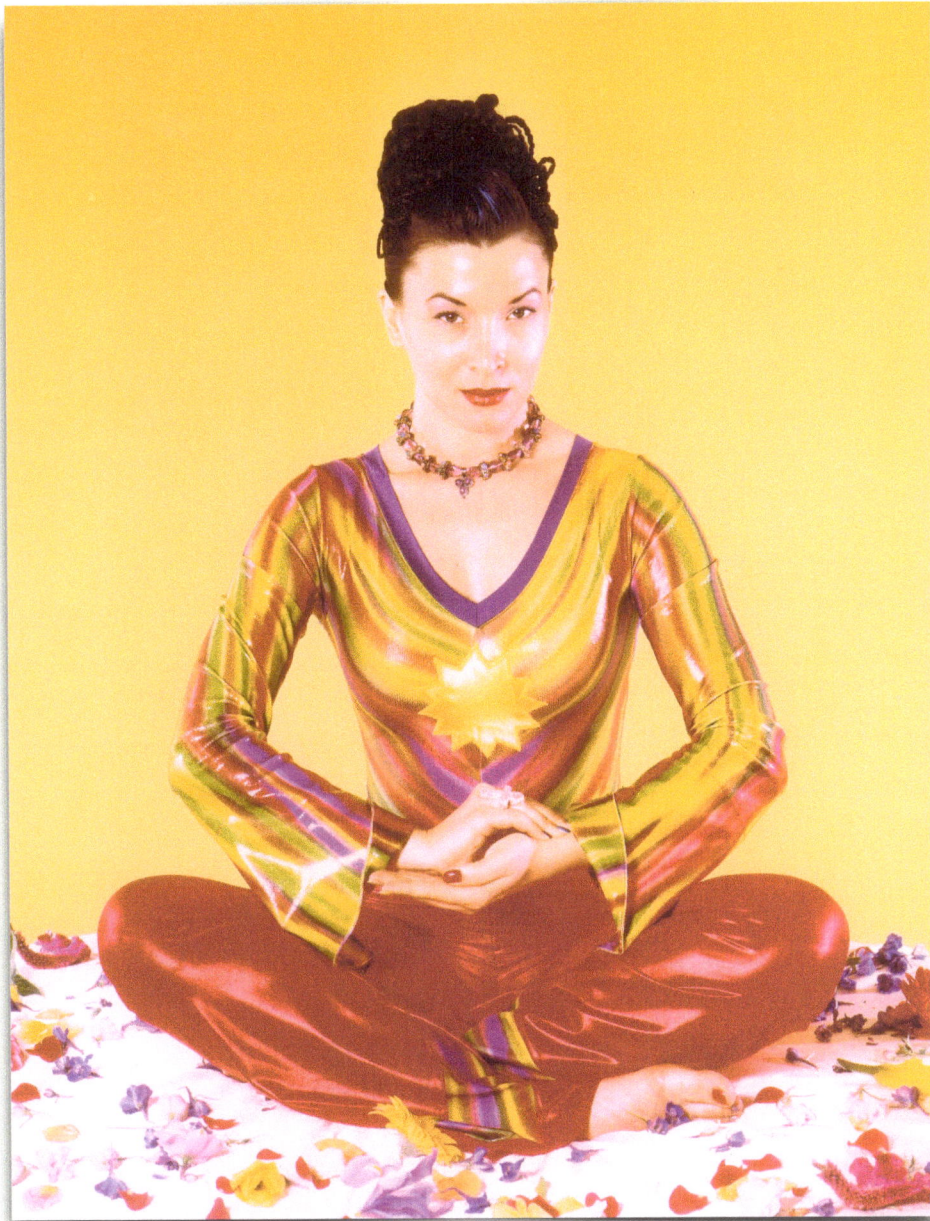

Sit with a straight back. With the four fingers of your right hand together in a straight line, feel the pulse on your left wrist. Press the fingers lightly so that you can feel the pulse in each fingertip. Palms are together. Close your eyes and concentrate on your Third Eye center.

BREATH: LONG, DEEP AND SLOW.

Practice this mudra for three minutes daily for a week.

MUDRA FOR GUIDANCE

Spiritual knowledge and wisdom have been given to every soul in this world. The answers to all of your questions are within your heart and are available to you at all times, twenty-four hours a day, including weekends, free of charge, no waiting list, credit check, or reservations required. You have the VIP seat. All you have to do is calm down, get centered, relax, ad use this mudra as the key to opening the door. Ask and you shall receive.

You receive energy and blessings into the palm of your hands.
Looking into them will send healing power to
Your mind and help you find guidance.

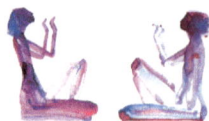

CHAKRA: Crown

COLOR: Violet

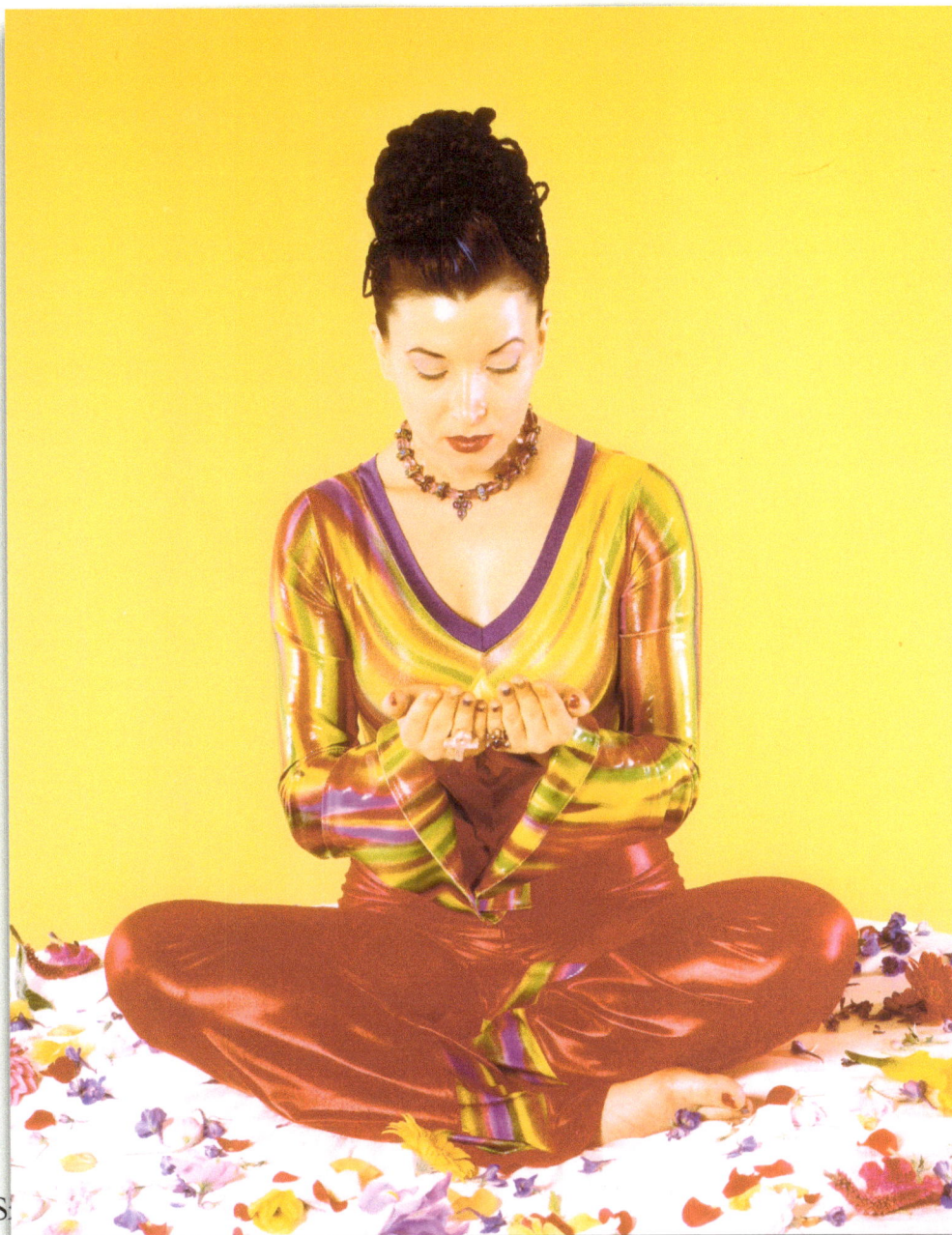

S[...]le fingers pressed together to form a cup with the palms facing toward the sky. Leave just a small opening between the sides of little fingers. Focus the eyes at the tip of the nose, toward the palms.

BREATH: LONG, DEEP AND SLOW INTO YOUR PALMS.

MUDRA FOR HELP WITH A GRAVE SITUATION

Sorrow and sadness can come upon us suddenly, and it is important that we know how to keep ourselves together in spirit, mind and body. Your heart is the center of emotion and love, and when an experience is particularly heartbreaking, you can actually feel physical pain in your chest and heart area. The healing power of your hands is used in this mudra to help you recharge, strengthen, and balance your heart and whole being.

This simple, ancient mudra will help you resolve any grave situation or conflict you are experiencing.

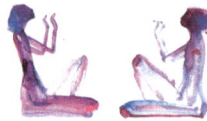

CHAKRA: Heart – 4

COLOR: Green

MANTRA: HUMME HUM, BRAHAM HUM, BRAHAM HUM
~ Calling upon Your Infinite Self ~
Repeat mentally with each breath

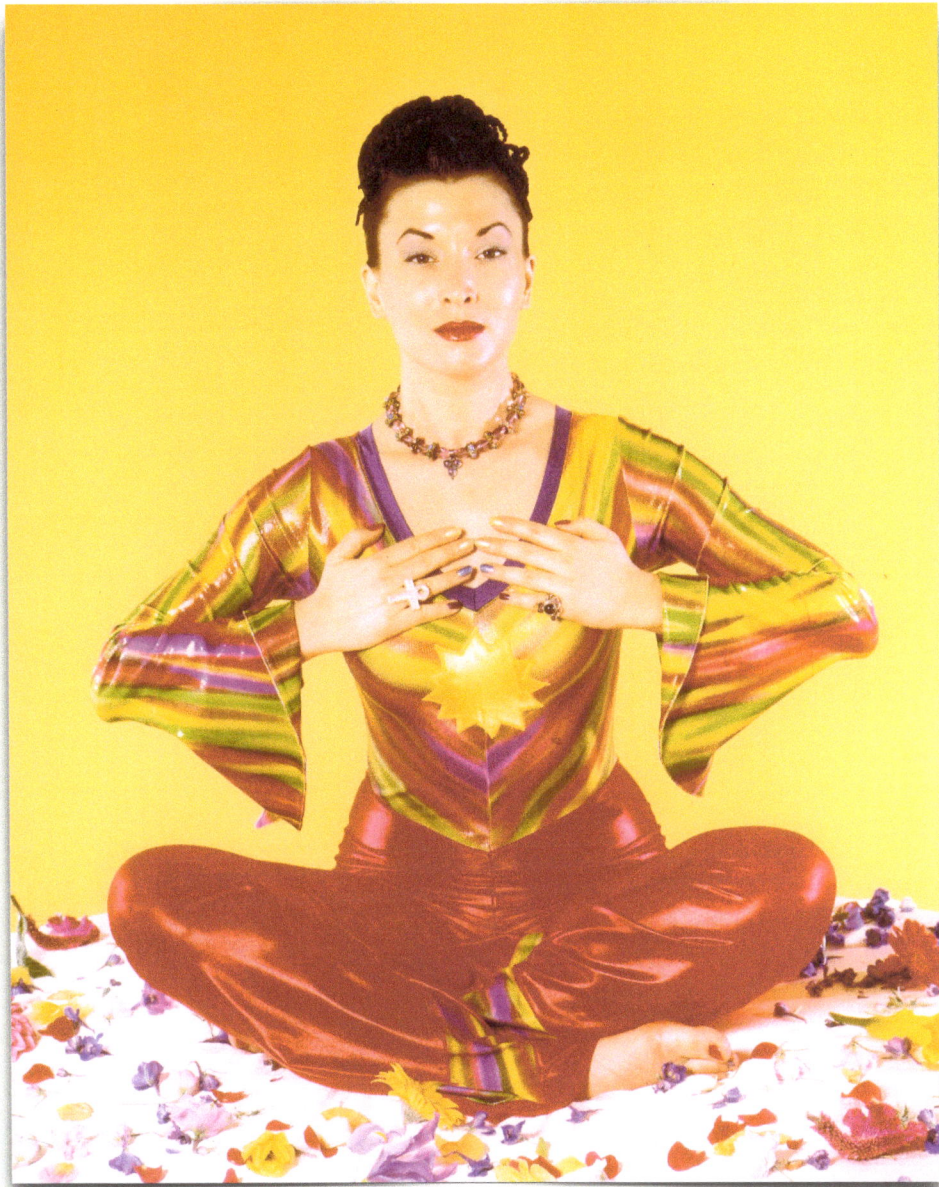

Sit with a straight spine. Place your palms on your upper chest, fingers pointing toward one another, elbows out to either side. The hands are relaxed with the fingers extended. This is a comfortable position with very little pressure and no tension in the arms and hands.

BREATH: LONG, DEEP AND SLOW.

Repeat a few times and notice calmness and peace surrounding you more each time.

Mudra for Powerful Insight

When you are unsure about what to do or how to remedy a problem, or you feel alone and confused, remember that you can find the answer within you. You just need to breathe deeply, calm down, and concentrate. With the help of this mudra, you will get the insight that you need. With regular practice, you will sharpen your intuition so that you may use it not only for yourself but also to help other people reach the same potential within themselves. We all possess the tools we need inside our souls.

This mudra coordinates both areas of the brain and Stimulates the insight centers.

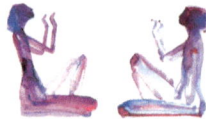

CHAKRA: Third Eye – 6

COLOR: Indigo

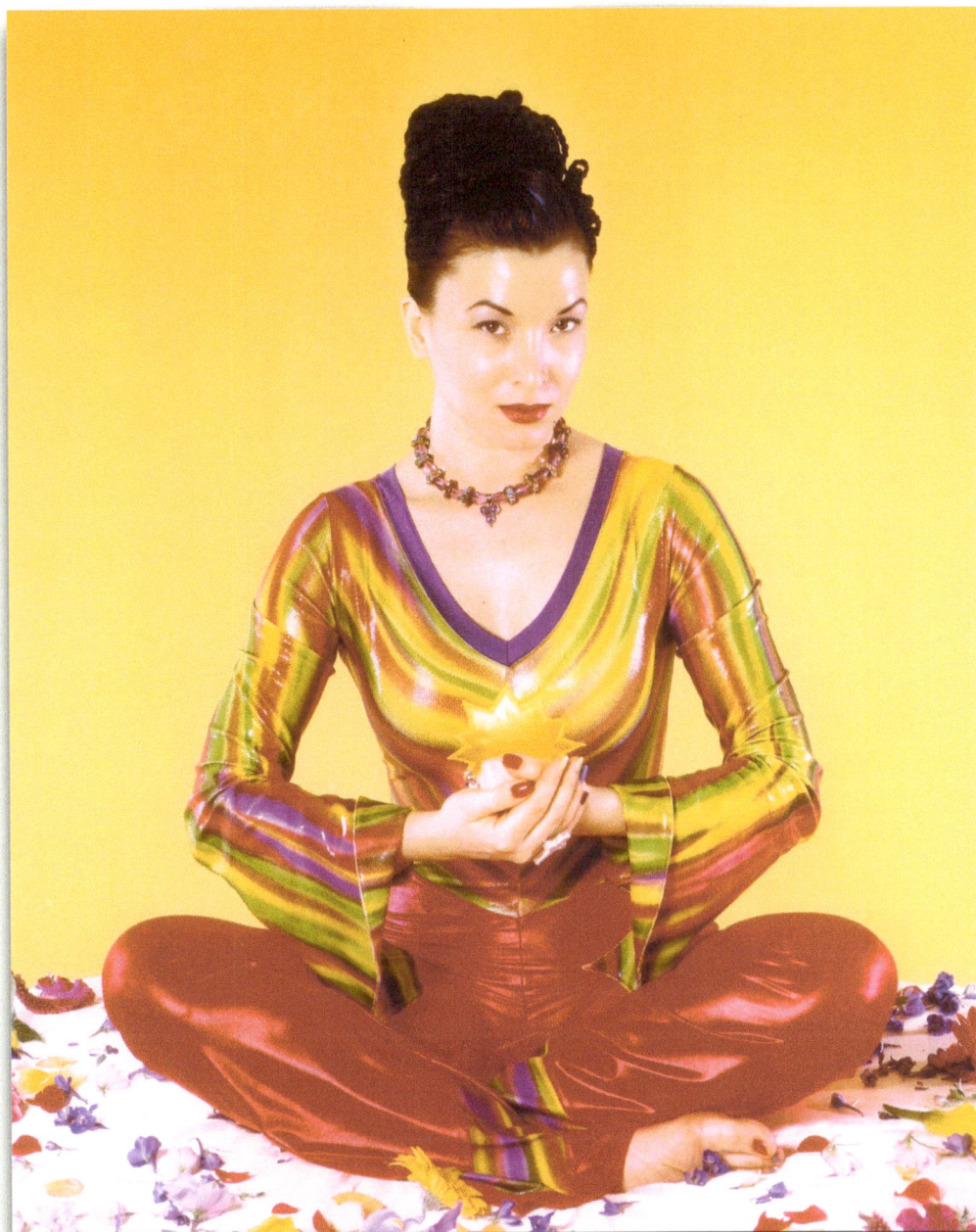

Sit with a straight spine, elbows out to either side. Raise your hands until they meet above the navel. The back of the left hand rests in the right palm and the thumbs are crossed, left over right. Concentrate on your Third Eye center.

BREATH: LONG, DEEP AND SLOW.

MUDRA FOR CONTENTMENT

We all experience unhappy moments, but sometimes we carry them with us longer than necessary. Living in the past affects your present and your future, so it is important for you to get to a place of serenity and contentment from which to view your life. A few minutes of this mudra will give you immediate results. A daily practice will transform your life.

This Mudra makes you feel cozy and content. The contact points between fingertips will redirect and balance your body energy and reinforce your inner ability to be in touch with your higher self.

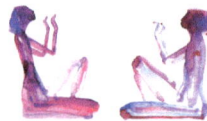

CHAKRA: Solar Plexus – 3
COLOR: Yellow

MANTRA: SARE SA SA SARE
SA SA SARE HARE HAR
~ God Is Infinite in His Creativity ~
Repeat mentally with each breath

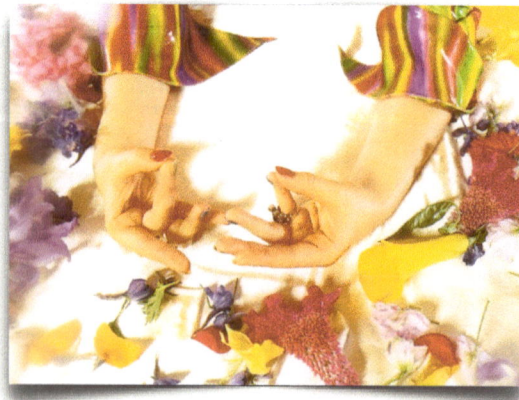

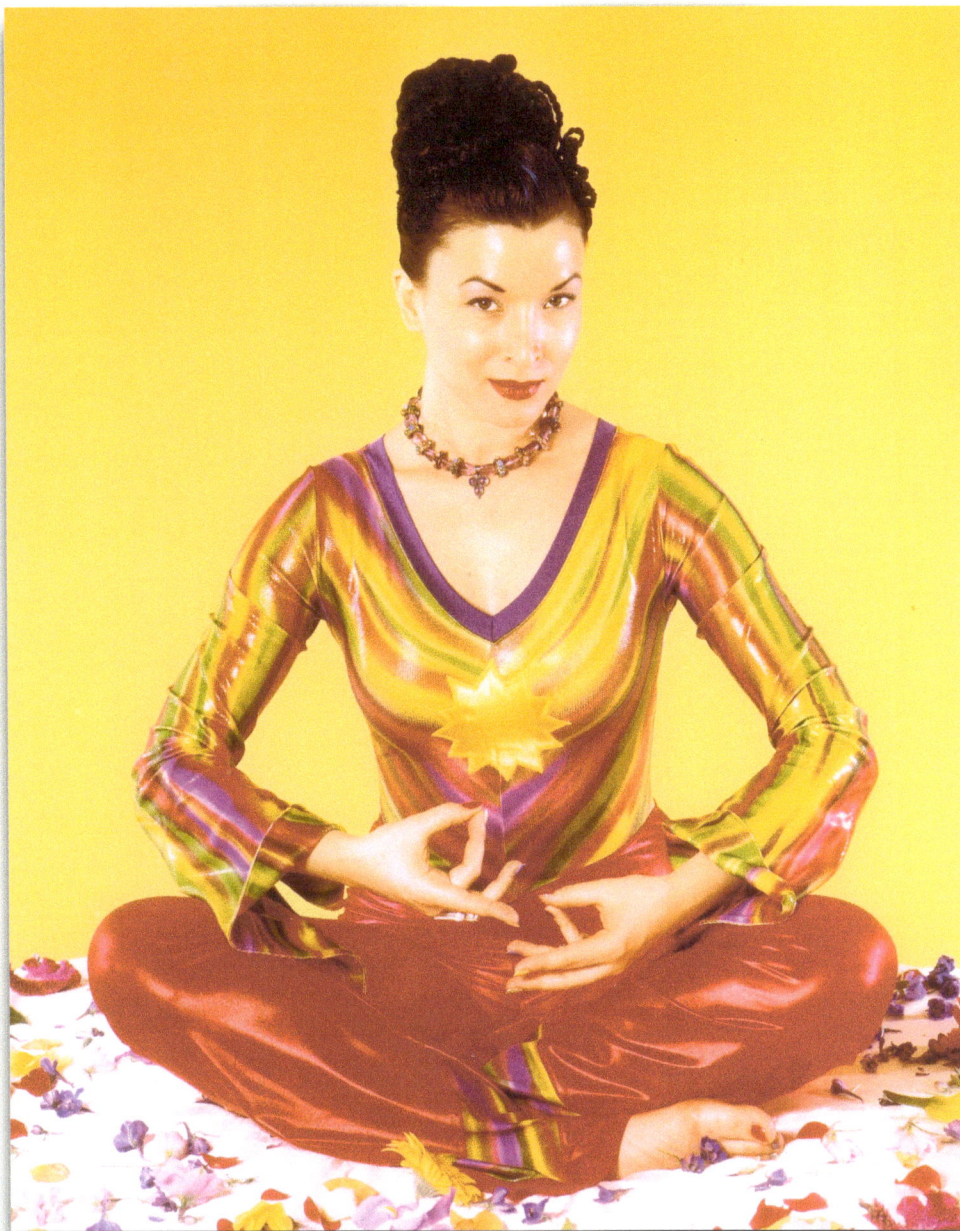

Sit with a straight spine. Make a circle with the thumb and middle finger of the right hand and thumb and little finger of the left hand. Relax but straighten the other fingers. Hold the hands a few inches apart in front of your navel area. <u>Men should make the same positions with opposite hands</u>.

BREATH: LONG, DEEP AND SLOW.

Meditate a few minutes, then make fists with both hands and relax.

MUDRA FOR PROSPERITY

Physical, emotional, and material prosperity is your birthright. How do you achieve it? First, have a clear goal and intention. See yourself successfully achieving and living your dream. Then, with this mudra, you rid yourself of any mental and emotional energy blockage in your past that stands in your way. Next, you must make practical, realistic plan of action. Practice with this mudra for eleven minutes every day for four weeks and see what happens. You should see your path clear and efforts rewarded.

You receive healing power into your palms with this motions of these hand positions. When you do this mudra with the chant "Har," you must and will manifest prosperity.

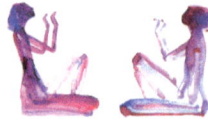

CHAKRA: Base of the Spine – 1
Reproductive Organs – 2
Solar Plexus – 3
COLOR: Red, Orange, Yellow
MANTRA: HAR HAR
(God, God)
Repeat loudly with each exhalation and hand movement, focus on the navel.

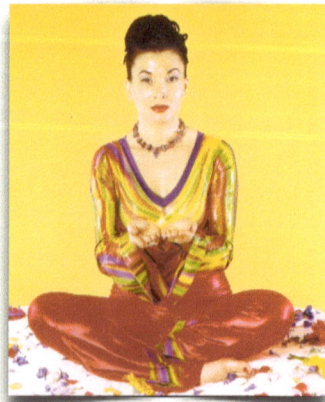

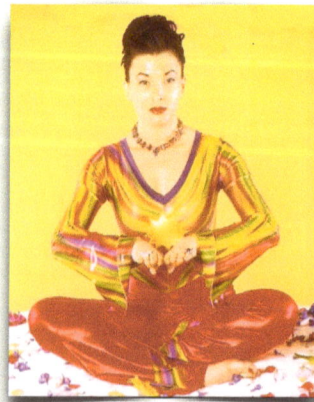

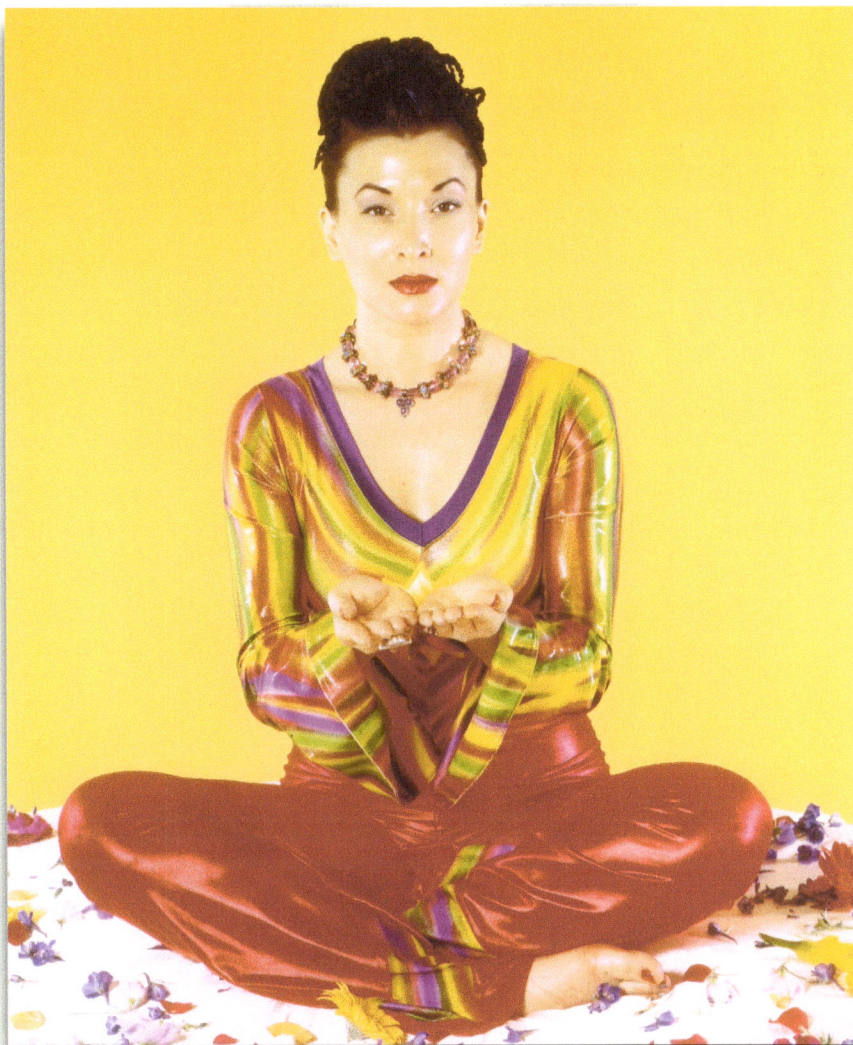

Sit with a straight spine and place the sides of your index fingers together, with thumbs hiding underneath the palms, palms facing the ground. Press the sides of the index fingers together firmly and hold for a second. Next, turn the hands over so the palms face the sky for one second, touching the hands together at the sides of the little fingers. Next, turn the palms toward the ground again, always keeping the sides of the hands touching. Each time you reverse the position of your hands, repeat the mantra "Har." Continue three to eleven minutes.

BREATH: SHORT, FAST BREATH FROM THE NAVEL. REPEAT THE MANTRA WITH EACH CHANGE OF HAND POSITION.

MUDRA FOR HIGHER CONSCIOUSNESS

Higher consciousness is the ultimate goal of your life's journey. We all long to be able to maintain a state of calm centeredness in the midst of daily storms, when everyone else is fighting confusion. All the answers are within you, available to you at all times, but to gain access to this inner power requires proper practice and discipline. It is up to you. Whenever you search consciously, you will find the answer you need. You've known it all along.

This mudra will help you achieve higher consciousness, deeper intuition, and increased spiritual strength — all of which will give you understanding of the hidden purpose behind everyday events and challenges.

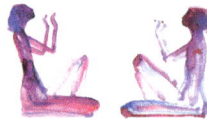

CHAKRA: Solar Plexus – 3
Crown – 7
COLOR: Yellow, Violet

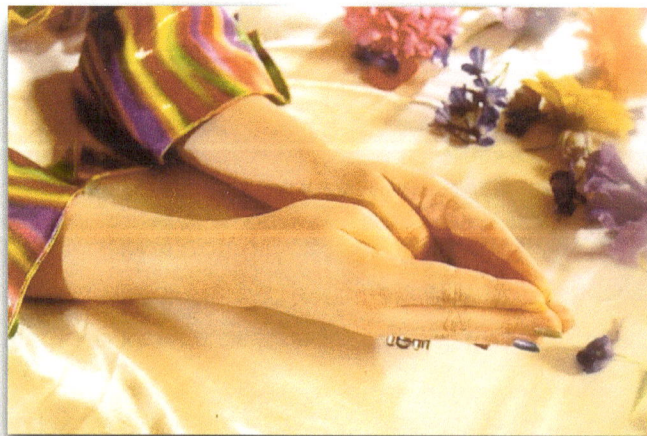

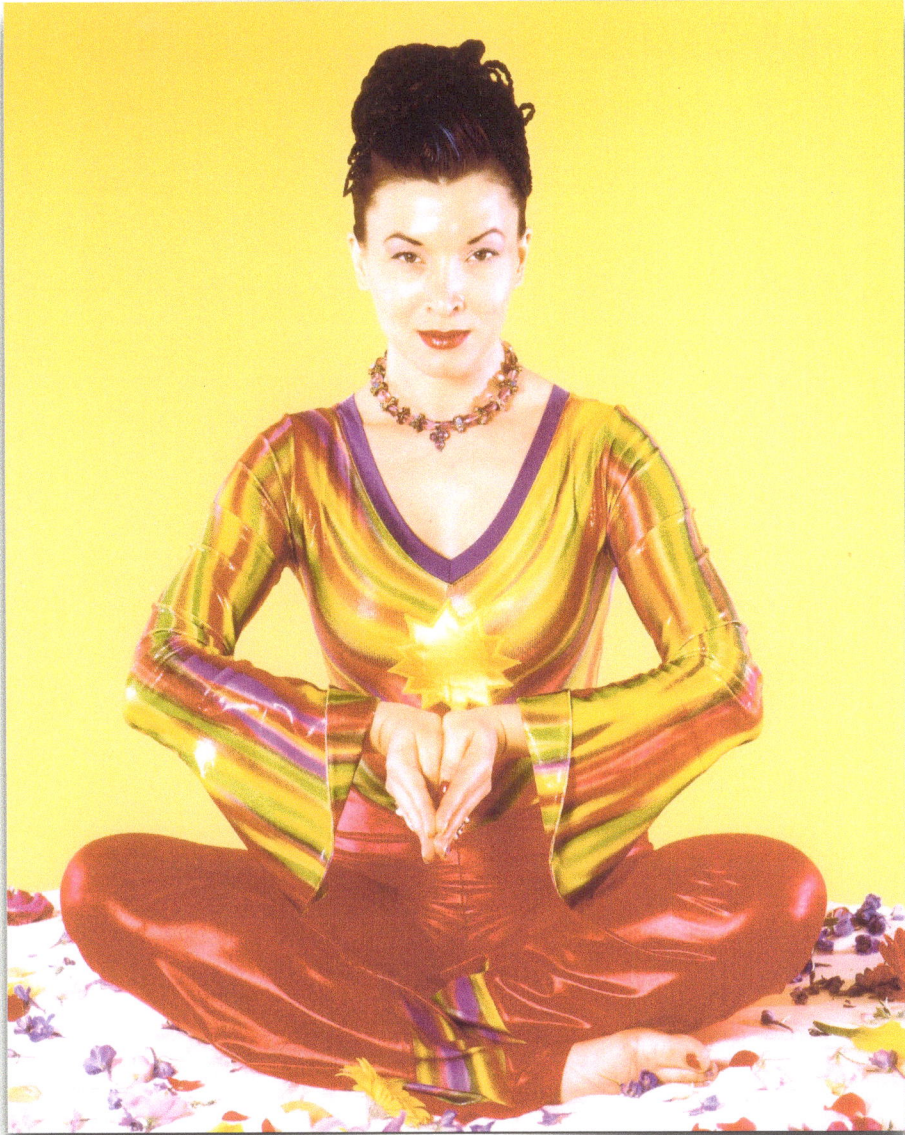

Sit with a straight back. Put your palms together, extend your elbows out to either side, and lift your hands in above your solar plexus area. Fingers pointed away from you. Each thumb is on the fleshy mound below the little finger of the same hand. Put the palms together, with the right thumb snugly above the left thumb. The bottoms of the hands touch firmly. Hold the hands a few inches away from the body.

BREATH: LONG, DEEP AND SLOW.

Repeat for a few minutes and build up your time. Relax and enjoy.

THE SACRED MUDRA SEQUENCE
FOR MENTAL, EMOTIONAL AND ENERGY BODY BALANCE AND CLEANSE

This very specific mudra sequence is called Kirtan Kriya. It is an excellent and effective tool to cleanse your Auric field and bring the mental, physical and emotional body into a state of balance. The pituitary and pineal glands are stimulated, the negative thought patterns can be erased and a new balance is established.

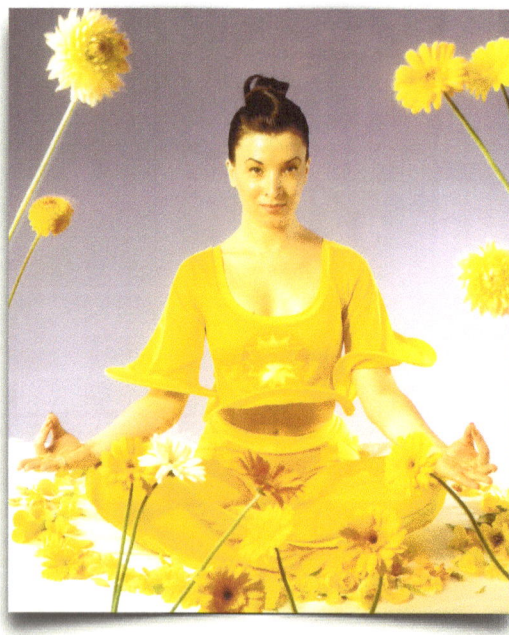

MANTRA:
SA TA NA MA
~ Infinity, Life, Death, Rebirth ~

Sit with a straight spine and rest the wrists on your knees. If possible stretch your elbows. Close your eyes and mentally focus on the area of the Third Eye. You will be connecting the thumb fingertips with other fingertips in a specific order sequence, while repeating the mantra.

TIMING:

THE MUDRA MANTRA SEQUENCE IS REPEATED AS FOLLOWS:

3 MINUTES IN NORMAL VOICE ~ awake state, earthly realm, the world

3 MINUTES IN LOUD WHISPER ~ longing to belong

6 MINUTES IN SILENCE ~ divine infinity

3 MINUTES IN LOUD WHISPER

3 MINUTES IN NORMAL VOICE VOLUME

These three modes of chanting relate to three levels of meditation:
With regular practice extend each segment to 5 min. and silence to 10 min.
Upon completion of this meditation sequence, deeply inhale and exhale,
stretch your arms up, spread your fingers, breathe long, deep and relax.

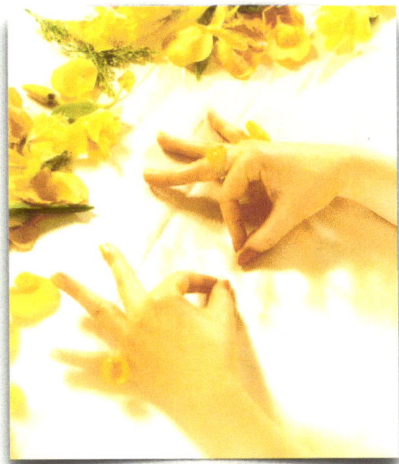

FIRST POSITION:
Connect and press together the thumbs
and index fingers while chanting: **SA**

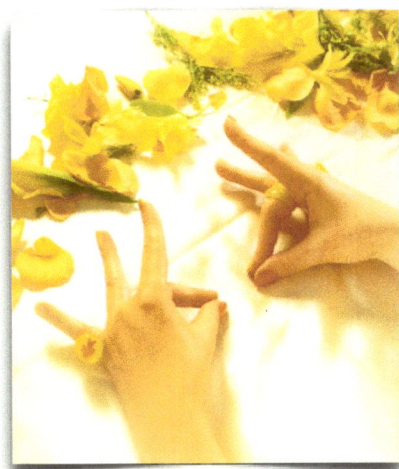

SECOND POSITION:
Connect and press together the thumbs
and middle fingers while chanting: **TA**

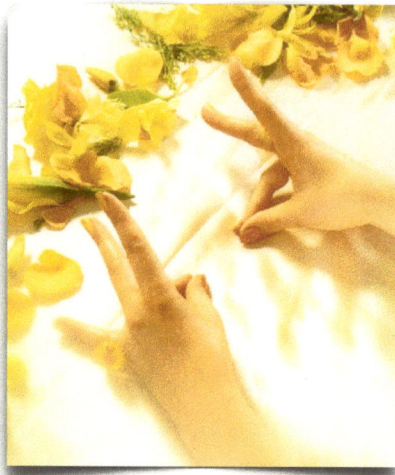

THIRD POSITION:
Connect and press together the thumbs and ring fingers while chanting: **NA**

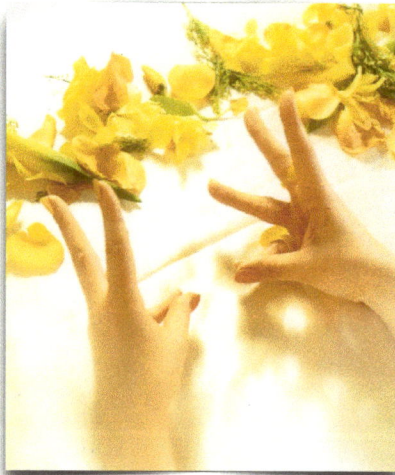

FOURTH POSITION:
Connect and press together the thumbs and ring fingers while chanting: **MA**

MUDRA INDEX

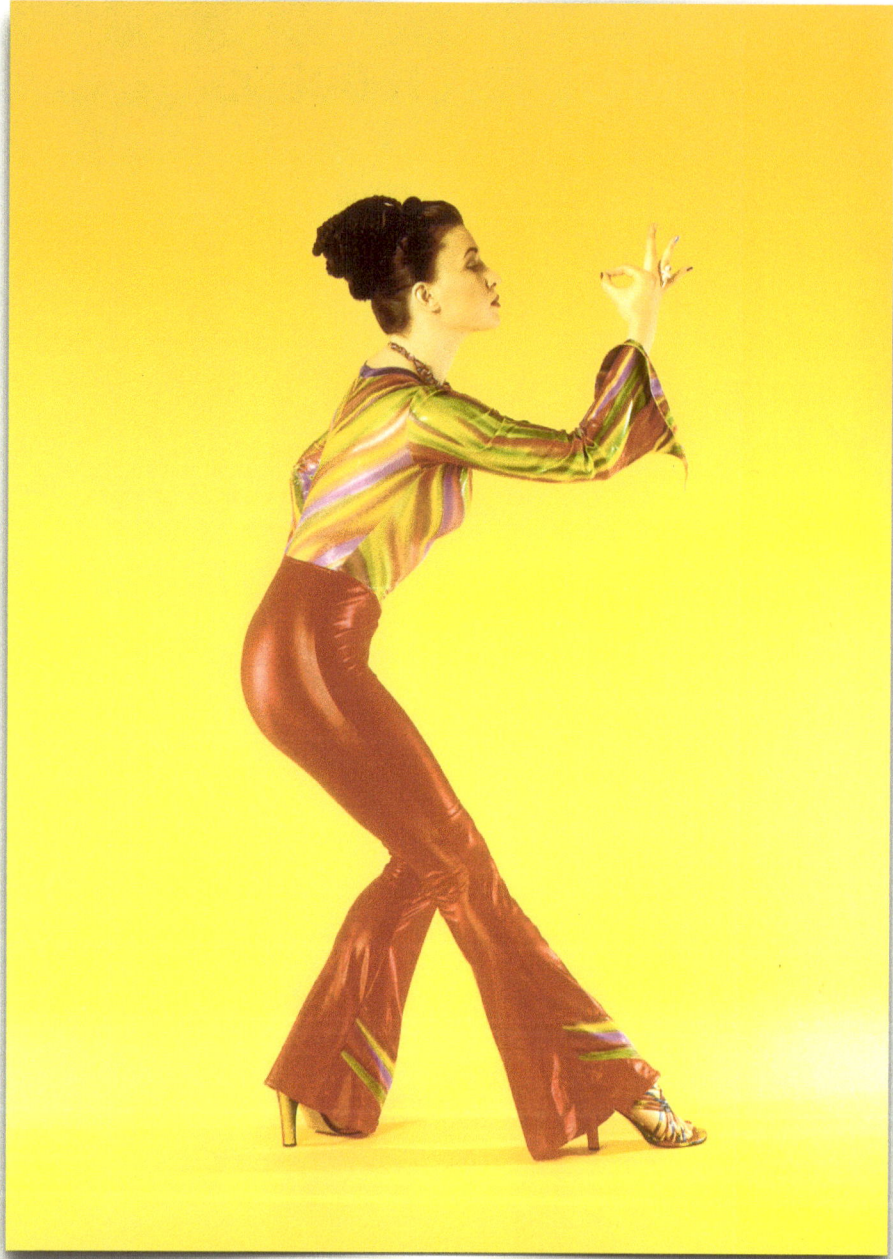

ABOUT THE AUTHOR

SABRINA MESKO   Ph.D.H. is a recognized Mudra authority and International and Los Angeles Times bestselling author of the timeless classic *Healing Mudras - Yoga for your Hands* translated into fourteen languages, as well as twenty other books on Mudras, Mudra Therapy, Mudras and Astrology, and meditation techniques.

Sabrina was born in Europe where she became a classical ballerina at an early age. In her teens she moved to New York and became a principal Broadway dancer and singer who turned to yoga to heal a back injury. She studied with Master Guru Maya, healing breath techniques with Master Sri Sri Ravi Shankar and completed a four-year study of Paramahansa Yogananda's Kriya Yoga technique. She graduated from the internationally known Yoga College of India and became a certified yoga therapist. An immense interest and study of powerful hand gestures - Mudras, led Sabrina to the Master who entrusted her with the sacred Mudra techniques giving her the responsibility to spread this ancient and powerful knowledge worldwide.

Sabrina holds a Bachelors Degree in Sensory Approaches to Healing, a Masters in Holistic Science, and a Doctorate in Ancient and Modern Approaches to Healing from the American Institute of Holistic Theology. She is board certified from the American Alternative medical Association and American Holistic Health Association.

She has been featured in media outlets such as The Los Angeles Times, CNBC News, Cosmopolitan, the cover of London Times Lifestyle, The Discovery Channel documentary on Hands, W magazine, First for Women, Health, WebMD, Daily News, Focus, Yoga Journal, Australian Women's weekly, Blend, Daily Breeze, New Age, the Roseanne Show and various international live television programs. Her articles have been published in world-wide publications. She hosted her own weekly TV show educating about health, well-being and complementary medicine. She is an executive member of the World Yoga Council and has led numerous international Yoga Therapy educational programs. She directed and produced her interactive double DVD titled *Chakra Mudras* - a Visionary awards finalist. Sabrina also created award winning international Spa and Wellness Centers and is a motivational keynote conference speaker addressing large audiences all over the world. Sabrina recently launched Arnica Press, a boutique Book Publishing House. Her mission is to discover, mentor, nurture and publish unique authors with a meaningful message, that may otherwise not have an opportunity to be heard.

She is the founder of MUDRA MASTERY ™ the world's only online Mudra Teacher and Mudra Therapy Education, Certification, and Mentorship program, with her certified graduates and therapists spreading these ancient teachings in over 28 countries around the world.

WWW.SABRINAMESKO.COM

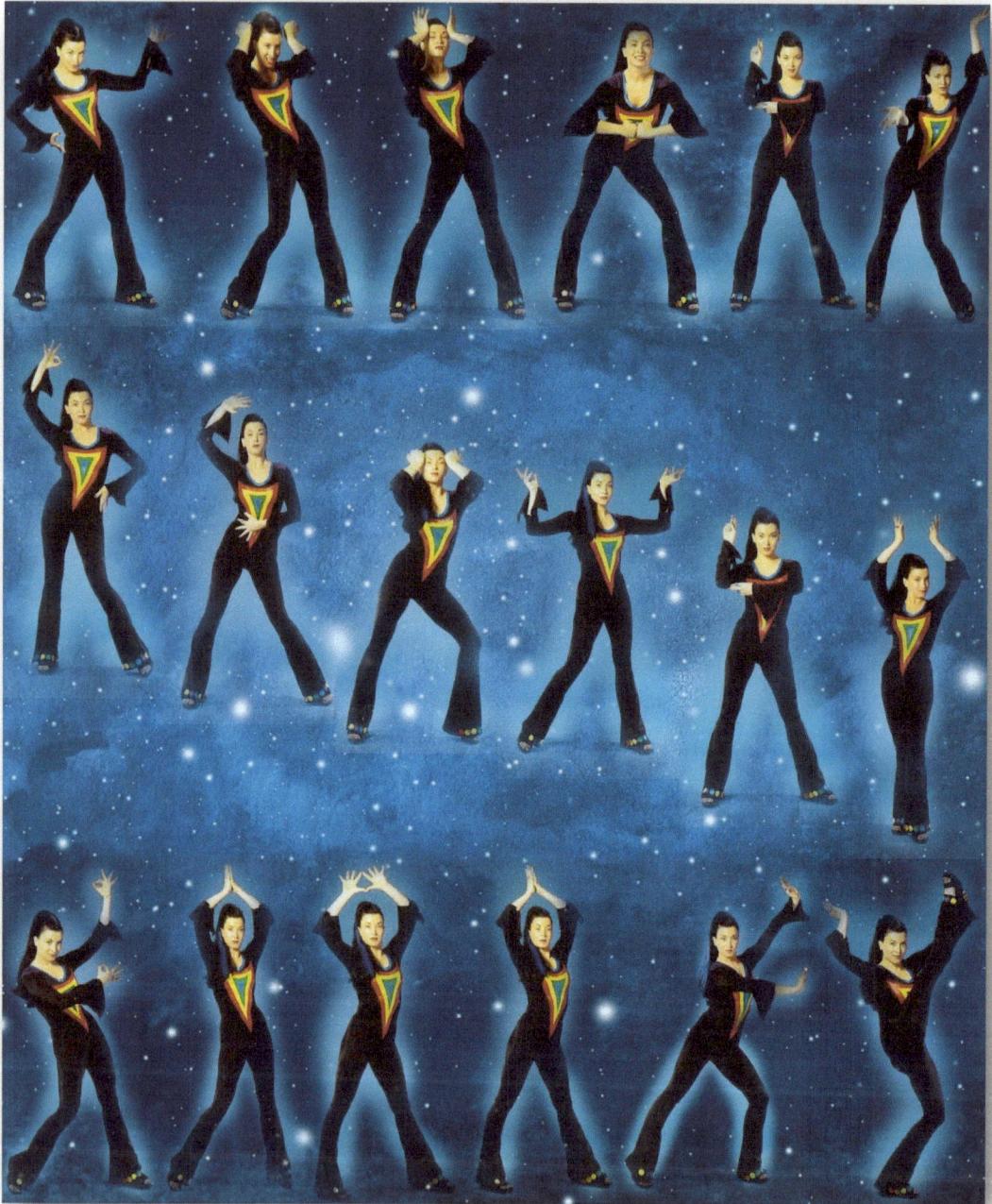

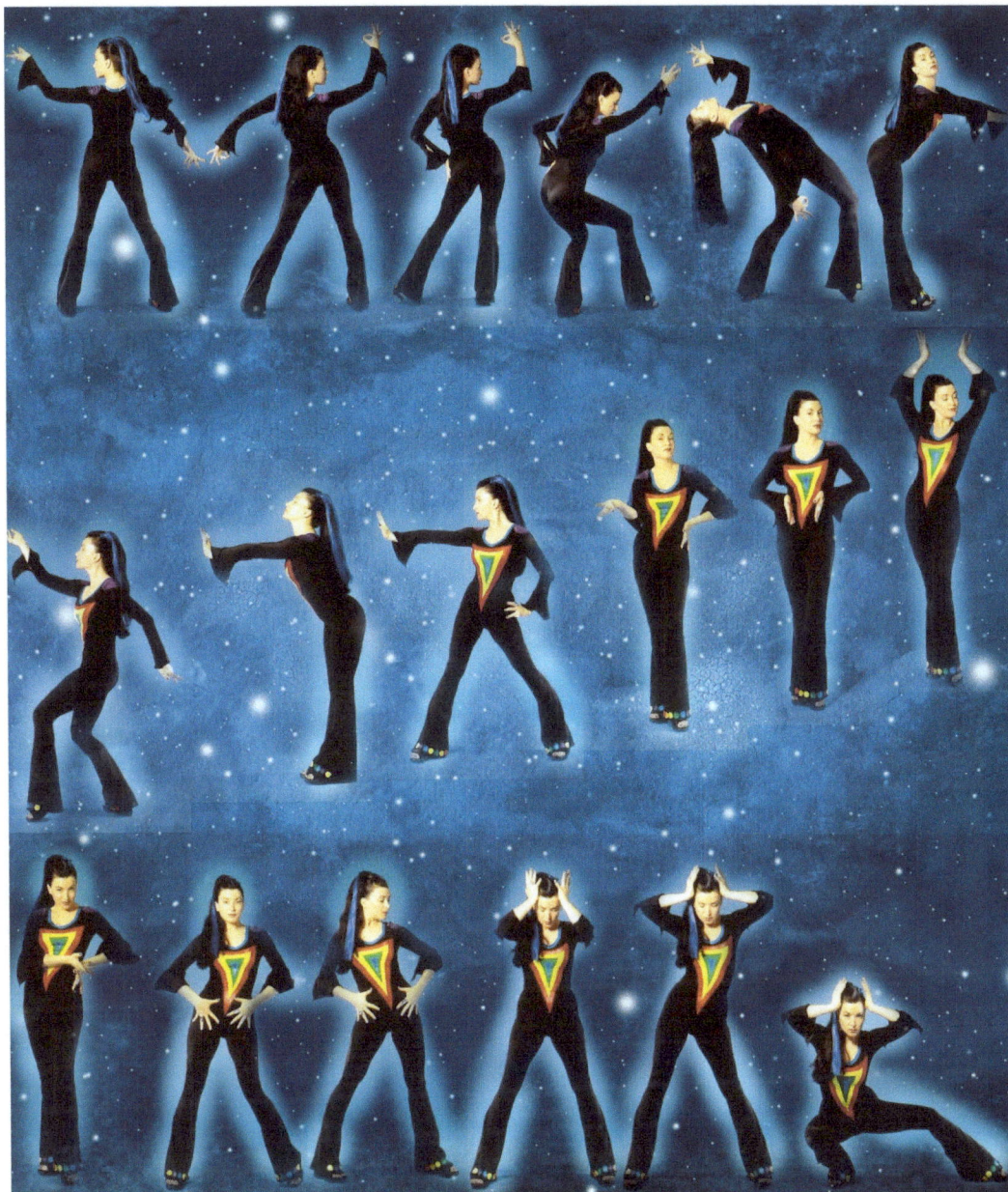

www.ingramcontent.com/pod-product-compliance
Lightning Source LLC
Chambersburg PA
CBHW060806270326
41927CB00002B/64